Home Remedies for Minor Health Problems

15 Common Health Issues and their Natural Cures

MARY CONRAD

ISBN: 1536843431
ISBN-13: 978-1536843439

DISCLAIMER

This book provides general information, personal experiences and extensive research regarding health and related subjects. The information provided in this book, and in any linked materials, is based on my own personal experience and is for informational purposes only. It is not intended to be interpreted as a professional medical advice. Speak with your physician or a trusted healthcare professional prior to taking any nutritional or herbal supplements. Please keep in mind that reactions and results may vary from each individual due to differences in state of health

Before considering any guidance from this book, please ensure you do not have any underlying health conditions, which may interfere with the suggested healing methods. If the reader or any other person has a medical concern or pre-existing condition, please consult with an appropriately licensed physician or healthcare professional. Never disregard professional medical advice or delay in seeking it because of something you have read in this book or in any linked materials.

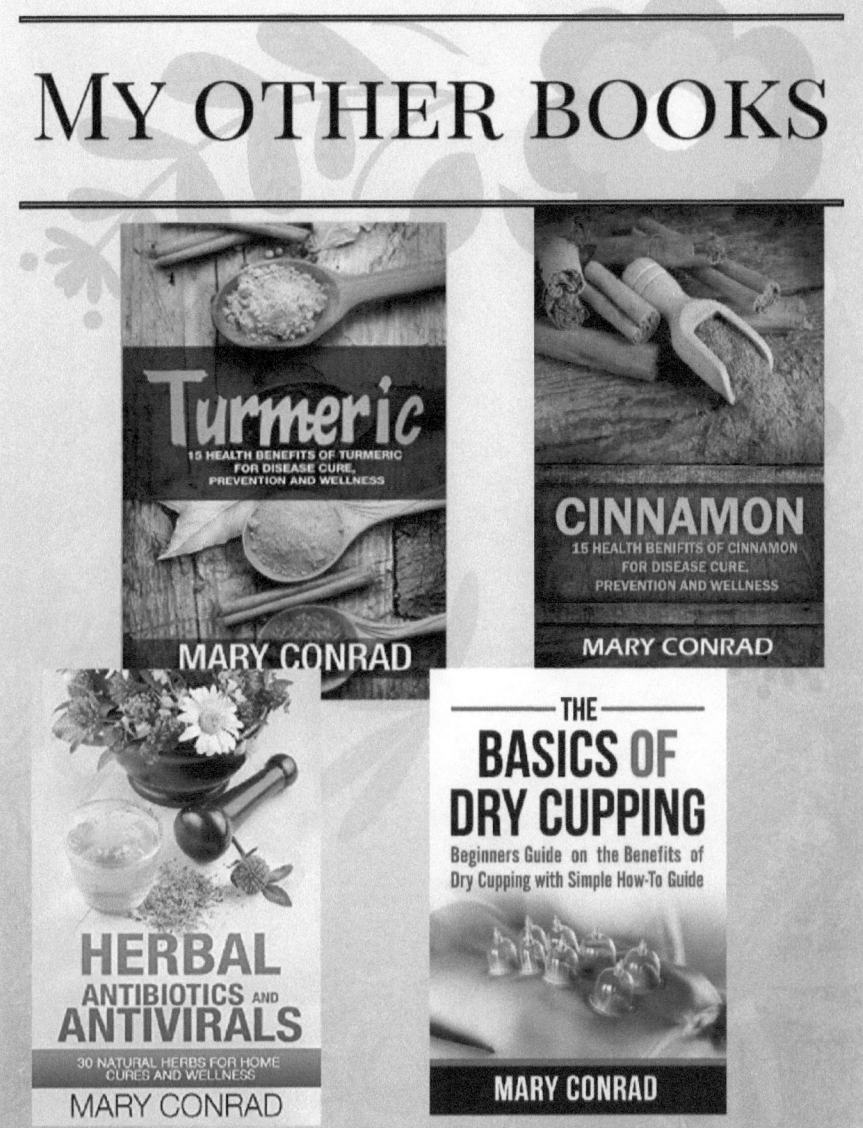

MARY CONRAD

CONTENTS

INTRODUCTION

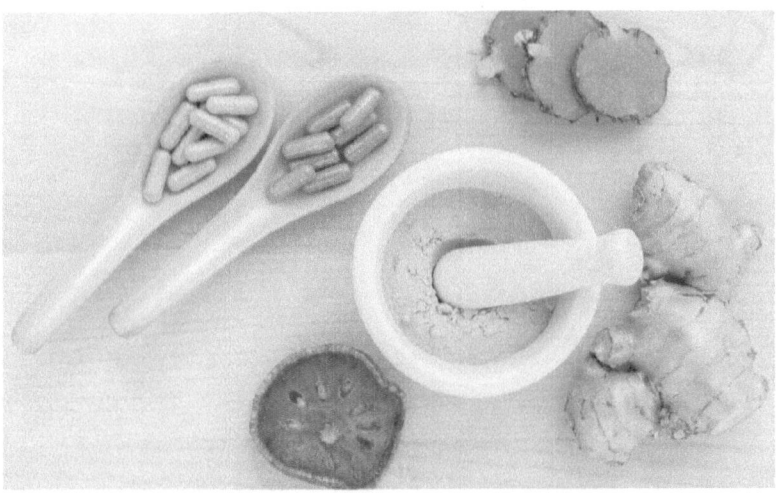

Minor health problems can be a bummer. I've had my share of everything from the sniffles to more serious complications of diarrhea. Being a nurse doesn't exempt me from being sick, I've actually had the most colorful health experiences throughout college. I've had multiple E.R. trips and one hospitalization over the course of four years. The great thing was my health problems cleared up after I got my diploma and learned how to take better care of myself without having to resort to taking strong antibiotics.

As a nurse, people expect me to give advice on the best pill to take when they're sick. Personally, my advice is to always seek professional help from physicians when the condition is moderate to severe, and when it impairs the normal activities of daily living. A physician is always the go-to for diagnosis and treatment for life threatening conditions.

For minor health issues, however, such as colds, flu, and diarrhea; there are home interventions and remedies that can be done safely without having to go to a physician. This is what I want to share in this book. Simple and practical interventions paired with some homemade remedies to assist sick family members to a healthy state without using pharmaceutical drugs. Although I may touch a bit about the use of herbs, most of the remedies that I will be discussing are with the use of common household items.

Take a step towards health today and let's take a journey to a better and more natural and healthy practices!

MARY CONRAD

Chapter 1

What is a minor health problem?

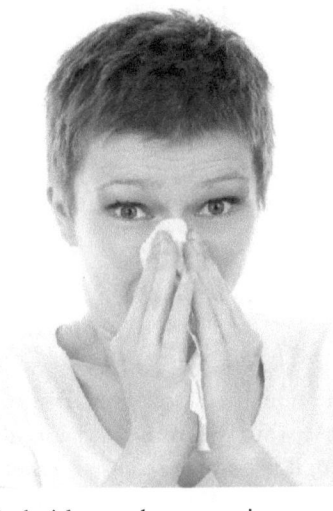

A minor health issue is a condition wherein there is a disruption in the normal bodily function, but does not require immediate medical assistance. These conditions are the type that can be addressed at home through over-the-counter medications or home remedies.

In the U.S. alone, there is approximately 14% - 27% non-emergency cases handled in the Emergency Room, resulting in long wait times when it could have been handled either at home or in outpatient clinics. For patients, it can result in frustration and poor quality of health service.

The advantage of treating minor health problems at home is that it saves you both time and money. For those who are more inclined to natural healing, an added advantage is better overall health.

When should you seek immediate medical help?

There are times when minor health problems can escalate into emergencies such as a when diarrhea results into severe dehydration or when allergies progress into an anaphylaxis or severe allergic reaction. The key is identifying when to seek medical help. Here are the danger signs to look for:

- Difficulty in breathing/shortness of breath
- Uncontrollable bleeding- bleeding that doesn't stop even when pressure is applied
- Impaired circulation - can be identified by bluish tinge on the lips, skin and nail bed
- Severe chest or stomach pain
- Excessive vomiting
- Persistent diarrhea
- Coughing up blood
- Disorientation
- Changes in vision, unexplained dizziness and body weakness
- Inability to stay awake
- Severe pain in any body part
- Sudden loss of ability to move or sensation in any part of the body
- Severe burns
- Deep puncture wounds (especially when there is no bleeding)
- Injuries in vulnerable areas such as eyes, spine and head
- Animal bites
- Fractures
- Severe allergic reaction wherein there is difficulty in breathing and severe swelling

These are just a few of the danger signs to look for. It's best to remember to always look at the ABCs or Airway, Breathing and Circulation. If there is a condition that affects the three, it is considered as an emergency and would need immediate assistance.

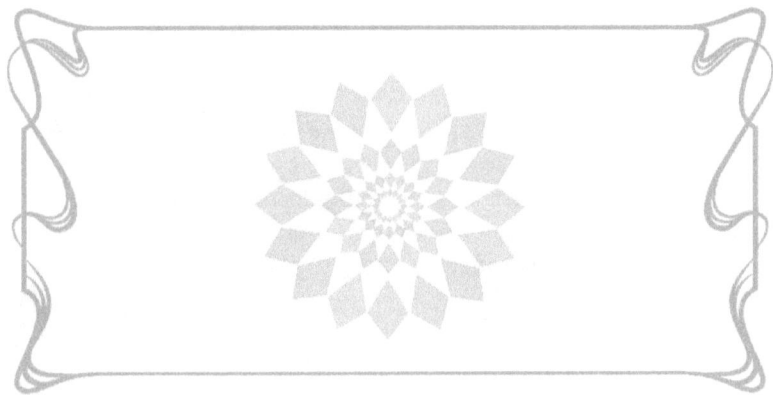

Chapter 2

The real deal on pharmaceutical self-medication

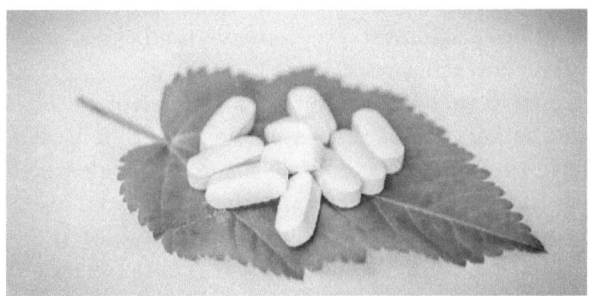

Self-medication is the act of using medicines without any advice from a professional to treat conditions that are self-diagnosed. Although there are some instances where self-medication is acceptable, such as when trying to relieve muscle pains or ease some discomforts from coughs and colds; the use of antibiotics without prescription is not something to take lightly.

The misuse of antibiotics can lead to drug-resistant infections. These types of infections would need to be fought with more potent antibiotics (broad spectrum) that target the infection in different pathways.

The risks for self-medication are as follows:

- Self-diagnosis, which may be incorrect.
- Treatment of symptoms may cause delay in proper treatment.
- Rare instances of severe reactions to self-medicated drug.
- Potential interactions from multiple drugs, such as maintenance medication mixed with nonprescription drugs.
- Lack of guidance in terms of drug administration, dosages and length of treatment.
- Possible misuse and abuse

A recent study has presented a possible solution, to address the common practice of self-medication. In any event wherein you're planning to self-medicate whether it is through drugs or home remedies, you either need to consult the pharmacist (for minor illnesses) or your trusted herbalist or holistic doctor. This is to ensure that there would be safety measures taken before self-medicating.

According to the World Health Organization, here are the responsibilities of your pharmacist, should you need assistance in responsible self-medication practices.

1. The pharmacist must recommend medicines based on proven safety, quality and efficacy.
2. The medicines recommended are for "self-recognizable" conditions, as well as diagnosed chronic conditions. The medication should have pamphlets that contain the dose and dosage forms.
3. The products need to have specific information that details:
   - how the medicine should be taken and used;
   - how the medicine works, and potential side effects;
   - how to monitor the effects of the drug;
   - potential interactions with other drugs or food;
   - length of treatment; and
   - when to consult a professional.
   - Keeping these in mind would go a long way to safely self-medicate.

Pharmaceutical medication isn't all bad and at the same time it isn't all good. It's merely a matter of using it correctly, knowing when to use it and how to take it properly. It is still evolving constantly to provide better treatment unlike the traditional methods of healing which have been around for eons.

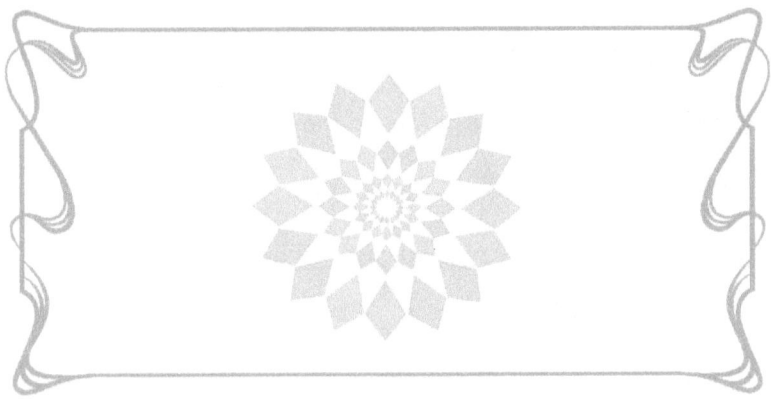

Chapter 3

Herbal Medications and Efficacy

Based on recorded history, the practice of herbal medicine has been around at least 3000 BC. From one of the oldest civilizations, such as China and Egypt, evidence suggests that the use of herbs and plants for healing was common. The most established forms of herbal healing are the Ayurverda and Chinese Herbal Medicine. Both of these are in practice throughout the world, and with the growing popularity of more natural approaches to healing, more and more people have become interested in the use of herbs.

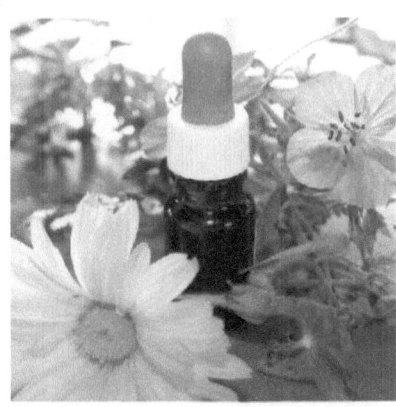

Most pharmaceutical drugs that we use today are derived from plants. It was around the 19th century when chemists and pharmacists began examining the chemical composition of plants to create the drugs that eventually became the mainstream line of treatment.

Does this mean that plants and

5

herbs are as effective as drugs? The answer is a resounding "Yes". There is still a big question as to why some herbs are more effective than drugs, but it is believed that the mixture of compounds in it may assist in increasing bioavailability. It is then metabolized in the body; yielding the desired therapeutic effect.

Herbs are just like the pharmaceutical drugs we have today, such as:

- It can be potent at certain dosages
- It can have side effects;
- It can lead to toxicity if taken with incorrect dosages;
- It can interact with other herbs; and
- It also has a recommended dosage.

There is always a safe and responsible way of taking medication, even herbs! Here are a few tips to take herbs safely:

- Do your research
- Get to know the herb you plan to use. Check for the therapeutic effect, side effect, contraindications and the danger signs to look out for.
- Check for herbalist or naturopath practitioner near your area
- A professional will be able to help you get the right therapeutic dosages for the herbs, and will be able to follow up on your progress.
- Find a local store that sells good quality herbs.
- Keep in mind that the better the quality, the better the results. It would be a great idea to find a trusted store so you're sure of the quality, even if it's a bit expensive.

Chapter 4

Cough

A cough is a reflex that helps clear out irritants and foreign bodies that enter the throat. It's one of the best mechanisms of mobilizing fluids in the upper respiratory tract and the throat to be removed through expulsion.

Since cough is usually a minor health issue, it is classified depending on its duration. An acute cough can last to about two to three weeks before it clears up on its own.

When a cough lasts between three to eight weeks, but shows recovery within the end of that period, it is classified as a sub-acute cough. This type can indicate a strong infection wherein the body is taking some time to fight it off naturally or through over-the-counter medications.

A cough that lasts for more than eight weeks is classified as a chronic cough. This can indicate a more serious health issue, and would need to be seen by a professional for diagnosis and treatment options.

Common Causes

Coughing is a symptom of an underlying health issue. It is the body's way of clearing out infection and secretions that can cause blockage of the airway and complications. Although coughing can be a bothersome thing, it is a form of defense mechanism that shouldn't be suppressed, unless necessary.

Here is a list of the common causes for cough:

- Acute Bronchitis
- Chronic bronchitis
- Colds
- Asthma
- Influenza
- Allergies
- COPD (chronic obstructive pulmonary disease)
- GERD (gastroesophageal reflux disease)
- Smoking
- Croup
- Intake of mucolytic medicines

Natural Remedies

For minor causes of cough, there are natural remedies to try out to relieve it. This is a great first line of treatment to avoid the unnecessary side effects of pharmaceutical medication.

There are different manifestations of cough such as a sore, itchy throat and chest pain from congestion. The remedies listed include ingredients that are common in your kitchen pantry, as well as some herbs that some of you might want to try out.

1. *Lemon and Honey*

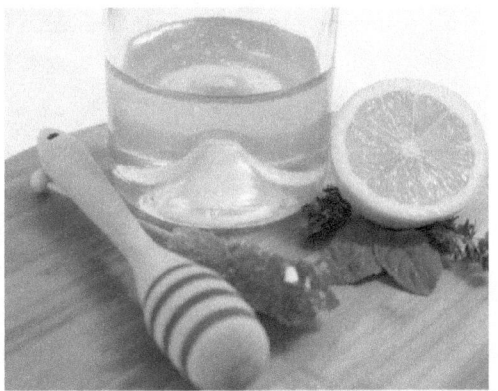

Lemons have numerous benefits in the body. The main compound, which is flavonoid glycosides, has some antibacterial and anti-inflammatory properties that help with fighting infections. The boost of vitamin C also helps in increasing immunity.

Honey has long been used to help soothe the throat, but a recent study done in 2007, showed that honey helps in suppressing cough. The subjects of the study were over 100 children and their parents. They were divided into three groups: one group of kids took honey prior to bedtime; the second group took a honey flavored dimethicone lozenge; and the third group were not treated. The results showed that honey had the same effect as the lozenge in suppressing cough.

Preparation:

A.) Lemon cough syrup:

Mix two tablespoons of fresh lemon juice and one tablespoon of honey. You can take this syrup several times daily as needed.

Note: Lemon can affect the enamel in your teeth. You may need to discuss this with your dentist prior to intake.

B.) Warm Lemon Juice and Honey

In a saucepan, boil about one cup of water. Pour 2 tablespoons of honey. Slice one whole lemon, and squeeze it over the honey mixture. You can drink this mixture as needed throughout the day.

C.) Lemon, Honey and Glycerin

For a raw and scratchy throat, glycerin is a great ingredient to throw in the usual mixture to help in moisturizing the throat.

1. Take a saucepan filled with water, and place a whole lemon to boil for 10 minutes.
2. Take out the lemon, slice and squeeze out the juice.
3. Add 2 tablespoons of honey, as well as glycerin.
4. Take one teaspoon once daily to relieve a raw and scratchy throat.
5. Store in an airtight container, and refrigerate for later.

D.) Lemon, Honey and Coconut Oil

Coconut oil is a great addition to your traditional lemon and honey blend. It is known to be rich in antioxidants and boosts immunity. With its many uses, coconut oil is a great staple in the kitchen.

1. In a saucepan, heat 2 tablespoons of coconut oil. Add 3 tablespoons of lemon juice and 1/4 cup of honey. Mix it well until the coconut oil has melted. Make sure not to boil the mixture.
2. Take one tablespoon daily until cough improves.
3. Store in an airtight container and refrigerate for later.
4. You may need to reheat this mixture once stored since coconut oil tends to solidify.

Precautions:

1. Honey can cause food poisoning in infants. Do not give honey to babies under 12 months or one year.
2. Before giving any of the remedies to a child, inform your physician to ensure safety.
3. Avoid using concentrated lemon for those with chronic heartburn or gallbladder disease.
4. If you're showing any signs of fever, shortness of breath, wheezing or difficulty in breathing, consult your physician.
5. It's always advisable to get diagnosed for the underlying cause of your cough.

2. *Carrot Juice*

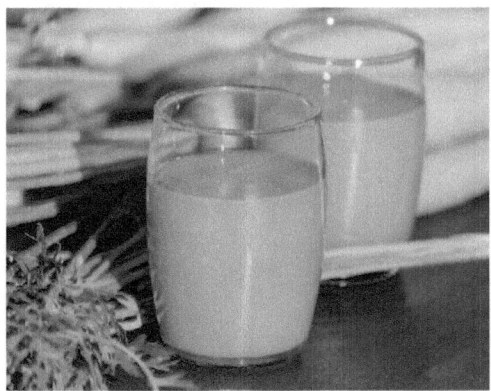

Carrots are rich sources of vitamins and minerals. It has antioxidant benefits that help prevent cardiovascular diseases, some types of cancer and cataract formation. As a cough remedy, carrots can help with dry cough. There has been little study in the benefits of carrots in relieving cough, but this vegetable has been in use for generations with great results.

A.) Carrot Cough Syrup

This is an old Portuguese recipe for dry cough.

1. Take one whole carrot, preferably the dark orange variety. Peel and cut into thin slices.
2. Place the slices in a glass bowl, completely lining the bottom. Sprinkle a thin layer of brown sugar.
3. Add another layer of carrots on top, and one last layer of brown sugar.
4. Let it sit uncovered for 12 hours or overnight.
5. Expect a dark syrup on the bottom of the bowl.
6. Take one tablespoon before meals and prior to bedtime.
7. Discard after two days.

B.) Carrot Juice and Honey

Make fresh juice from four to five carrots and add some water to dilute it. For taste and added benefits, add one teaspoon of honey.

Drink the juice three to four times a day until your symptoms improve.

Precautions:

Vitamin A isn't meant to be consumed at high dosages. It's very rare that diet can lead to toxicity. A sign that you may have had too much carrots is a slight yellowing of the skin, which is especially prominent on the hands. You may need to cut back on the intake once this occurs, but it is generally harmless.

3. *Turmeric*

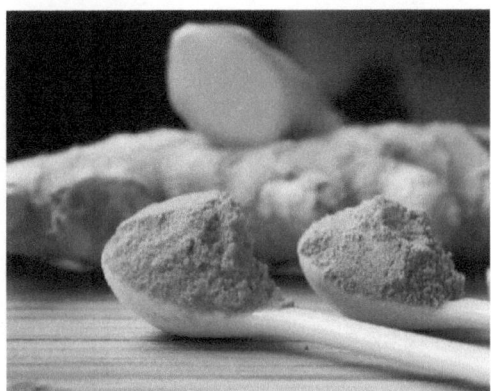

Turmeric is known for its anti-inflammatory properties. The active ingredient, which is curcumin, helps on reducing chest congestion from inflammation. This spice offers relief for dry cough.

Preparations:

There are several ways to use turmeric in relieving cough.

A.) In a small pot of boiling water, add some ground turmeric and black pepper. The amount is as per tolerated, adjust according to your preference. Pour a tablespoon of honey. Let the mixture cool. You can add some ground cinnamon for a comforting aroma. Drink this solution once daily until your cough improves.

B.) For chronic cough, boil a mixture of goat's milk. Add about 1-2 teaspoons of turmeric (or as tolerated). Add a pinch of black pepper to aid in absorption. Let it cool and drink.

Although there are a few more ways to prepare turmeric for cough, these two are the easiest to prepare and well tolerated. For those who want to prevent the recurrence of coughs that are caused by inflammation, you can take the turmeric and milk mixture as a preventive measure.

You can also check out my book on turmeric for more recipes and information on the spice.

Precautions:

1. For those who will undergo any surgery, avoid taking turmeric for two weeks prior to surgery, since it acts as a blood thinner and can cause bleeding problems

2. Those who have gall bladder problems, kidney disease, ulcers, and immune system issues, consult a physician prior to taking the spice as it might interact with maintenance medication or aggravate the symptoms of condition.

4. *Grapes*

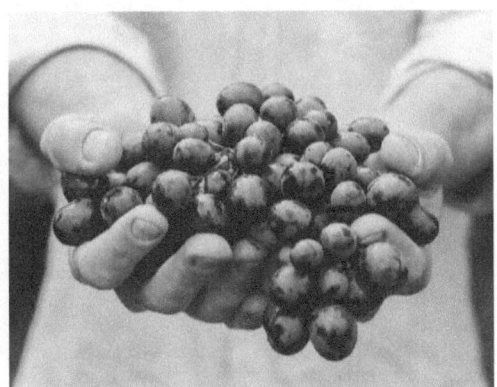

Grapes is a rich source of vitamins, minerals and antioxidants, but it has shown to have significant effects on the lungs and respiratory system.

Grape seed extract, which is obtained from the seeds of red grapes, has proven to be effective in improving lung function. According to a study in 2011, it has shown to lower airway resistance, reduce the number of inflammatory cells and decreases the goblet cells in the airway. The goblet cells are responsible for mucus production. The decrease in inflammation and reduction of mucus production, helps in facilitating its removal from the airways which stops the coughing.

Preparation:

A.) Grape Juice
  1. Toss in fresh grapes into a blender
  2. Add a teaspoon of honey
  3. Blend until smooth.

C.) Fresh Grapes
  Pop a grape in your mouth and enjoy!

5. *Ginger*

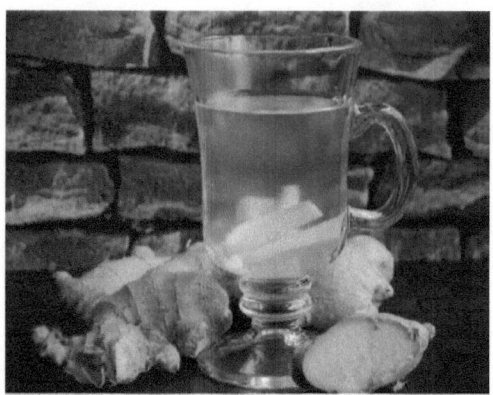

Ginger is one of the most popular natural cures for a cough. With its antibacterial properties, it can help ease the condition by addressing the underlying cause of the cough. Oleoresin is a chemical component found in ginger that acts as a cough suppressant. This spice also has other phenolic compounds that mainly affects the gastrointestinal system, and is believed to be the reason behind the medical properties of the root.

A.) Ginger Tea

This tea is great for chronic cough and sore throat.
1. Peel and cut ginger into small slices.
2. Lightly crush the small pieces to release the juice.
3. In a saucepan, add one cup of water.
4. Toss in the ginger slices and bring to a boil.
5. Add a teaspoon of honey and lemon juice to boost the flavor.
6. Drink three times daily for symptom relief.

B.) Raw Ginger

This is great for dry cough and those who don't mind the strong flavor of ginger.

1. Peel and cut a small slice of fresh raw ginger.
2. Chew it periodically throughout the day

Precautions:

1. In small dietary doses, ginger may cause gas, heartburn, upset stomach and irritation of the oral cavity. The larger the dose, the more likely the

side effects occur.

2. For pregnant women, those with diabetes, or any heart problems, you may need to check with your physician prior to taking moderate to high doses of ginger.

6. *Almonds*

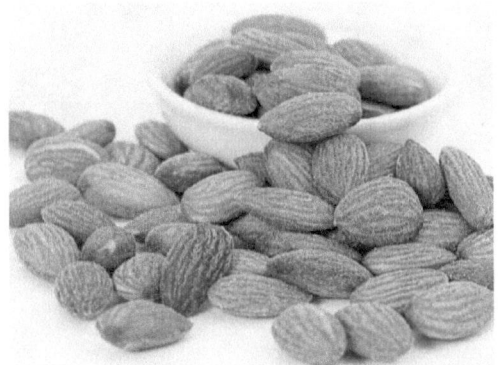

These nuts have nutritional properties that play a proactive role in healing cough symptoms. It is also highly nutritious.

Preparation:

A.) Almond Butter

1. Soften five to six almonds by soaking them in water for 8-10 hours.
2. Ground the almonds into a paste.
3. Add one teaspoon of butter
4. Take the paste three to four times daily until cough is relieved.

7. *Garlic*

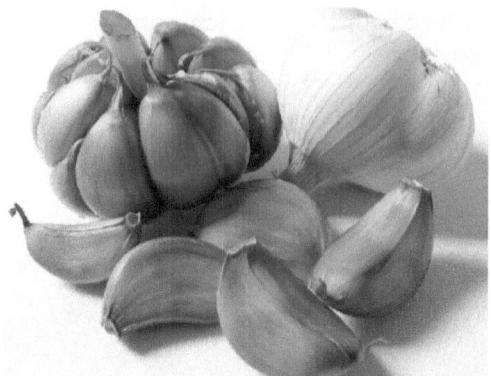

Garlic has antibacterial properties that aid in treating cough by killing the infection. It helps aid your body in fighting off the pathogens and also by boosting immunity.

A.) Raw Garlic

Eat crushed raw garlic. You can add a bit of honey for relief from sore throat.

B.) Garlic Tea

Take three cloves of garlic, crush it. Add it into a cup of boiling water. Toss in about a teaspoon of oregano. Strain the mixture. Let it cool. Pour some honey and drink it.

8. *Pineapples*

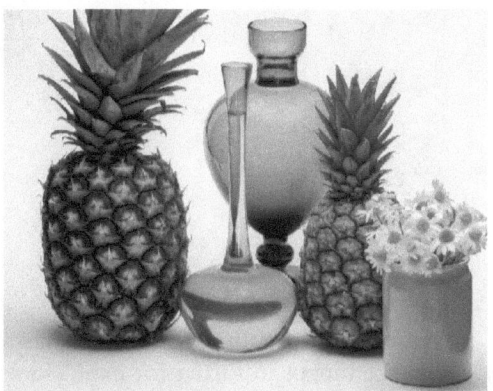

This tropical fruit is rich in vitamins and antioxidants. An enzyme found in this fruits, bromelain, contributes to its great effects on cough and immunity. It not only suppresses cough but helps in mobilizing thick secretions that are in the throat. Removing the irritants will stop the cough.

Preparation:

A.) Eat the fresh fruit
B.) Drink pineapple juice.

Precautions:

Bromelain supplements should not be taken in conjunction with antibiotics. There is a potential for drug interactions. It also enhances absorption. Those who take blood thinners should also be careful before consuming supplements and increasing dietary intake.

Children, nursing and pregnant women should also avoid supplements, unless indicated by a doctor.

Peppermint and Eucalyptus

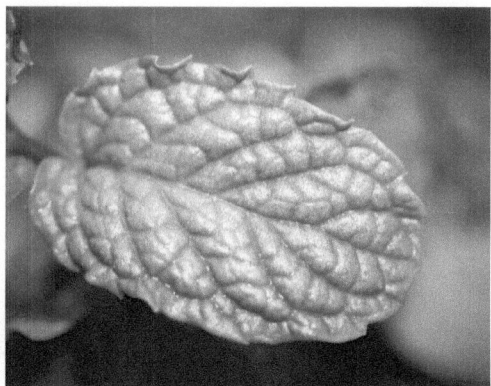

Peppermint leaves contain menthol, which helps soothe the throat. It also helps break down the mucus in throat for expulsion.

Preparation:

A.) Peppermint tea

You can use prepackaged peppermint tea or make your own.

1. Gather fresh mint leaves and wash it thoroughly. Set aside.
2. Boil about one cup of water. Once done, pour the water in a cup.
3. Add the mint leaves and let it steep for five to ten minutes.
4. Remove the leaves. Add the sweetener of your choice.

**For dried peppermint leaves, allow it to steep for 10-15 minutes. Drink this three times daily until relief is felt.

Tip: You can add a different flavor by adding lemons while the tea is cooling or vanilla beans.

B.) Peppermint vapors

1. Add three to five drops of peppermint oil in a large bowl of hot water (150 ml of water per drop of oil).
2. Prepare a towel beside the bowl.
3. Lean towards the steam and vapor, making sure to keep a safe distance from the hot water.
4. Cover your head with the towel.
5. Do this for about 15 minutes.

Eucalyptus oil

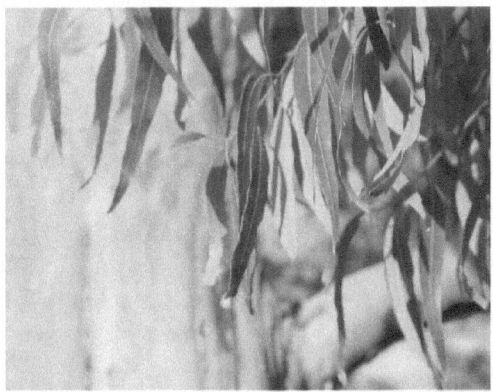

Eucalyptus oil has been used for centuries as a cure for respiratory problems. It provides relief from congestion either by application on the skin or through inhalation of vapors.

A.) Eucalyptus rub

- 1/2 cup of coconut oil
- 1/4 cup of beeswax
- 10 drops of eucalyptus oil

Heat the beeswax in low heat until melted. Add the coconut oil and stir well. Take out of the heat and let it cool a bit before adding the eucalyptus oil. Stir well then transfer into an airtight container.

You can store this at room temperature for 12 months.

Precautions:

Eucalyptus and Peppermint essential oils are not safe for young children to use. Peppermint oil should not be used for children under six years of age. Eucalyptus is not to be used for children under 10 years of age. This goes for both skin applications and diffusion.

Home Intervention

There are techniques where you can manipulate the body into expelling the secretions. During community health nursing, some of these techniques were taught in order to assist those who require it as well as educate the family members on how they can do it safely at home.

Here are the three basic massage treatment to help mobilize secretions:

1. As the patient to sit on a chair without a back rest.

2. You can use the eucalyptus rub for maximum effect. Apply the rub on the person's back.

3. Start by effleurage to help the person relax. Using the palms, apply even pressure throughout the back. Move your hands in a downward-upward-outward motion. The movement needs to be synchronized. Do this for five to ten minutes.

4. Next massage is tapotement, this is a group of massage that involves cupping, hacking, pounding, pummeling and tapping. This movement helps in loosening secretions. The pressure should be even and firm but not so strong as to cause tissue damage. For this technique, you need to take a few precautions such as avoiding bony prominences.

   This is not to be used for:
   • Pregnant women
   • Over nerves
   • To paralyzed individuals

5. The last massage is petrissage, this involves kneading, rolling, lifting and wringing. This is a great technique to help the tissues eliminate any waste products while improving the muscle tone.

   This is not advised for:
   • Those who have recent damage in the skin or muscles in the area
   • Pregnancy
   • Hernia

6.   Close off the massage with a relaxing effleurage.

Note: If in doubt, always consult a trained professional. They can help assist you and will provide the services with your safety as a primary concern.

When to see a doctor

Cough usually clears out in a week or two without any problems but if you develop fever, wheezing and experiencing shortness of breath; this could indicate a serious infection. Bloody or green mucus secretions also indicate infection and immediate medical assistance is required.

MARY CONRAD

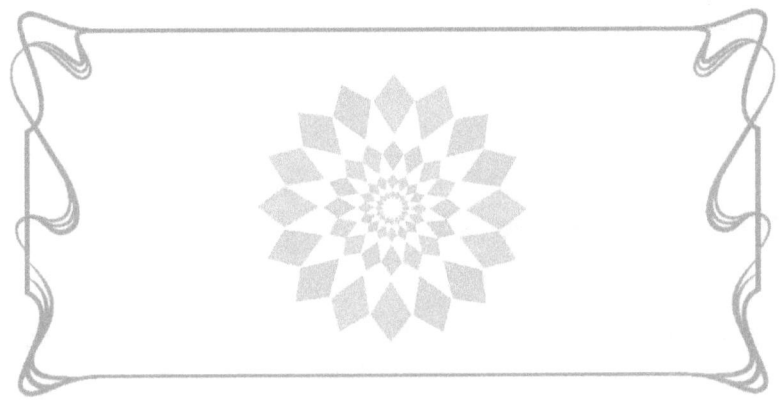

Chapter 5

Cold

A cold is a viral infection that is usually just mild and goes away on its own. It initially starts with a sore throat for a day or two followed by a runny nose. The secretions are usually clear at this point. After a few days or about a week, cough will begin to develop from post nasal drip and the secretions will be darker and might turn into a yellowish green hue.

Colds usually clear out within a week or two for adults. In severe cases, it can cause a mild fever and sinus headaches. For children, fever is more common but usually this also clears out once the symptoms begin to show. The virus spreads more rapidly in the first three days of infection.

Influenza or "flu" is caused by a different virus. It's a bit more severe compared to colds and can take weeks before clearing out. There are several differences between the two in terms of symptoms but it can easily be interchanged. Flu symptoms include colds, fever, headache, muscle aches and soreness, fatigue and cough.

After a week, flu symptoms often lessen but feelings of fatigue can take weeks to subside. Although flu seems common enough, it can have severe complications such as pneumonia, which can be fatal for the elderly, infants and those who have low immunity.

In cases where difficulty in breathing is experienced, seek medical attention.

Natural Remedies

1. Spice Tea

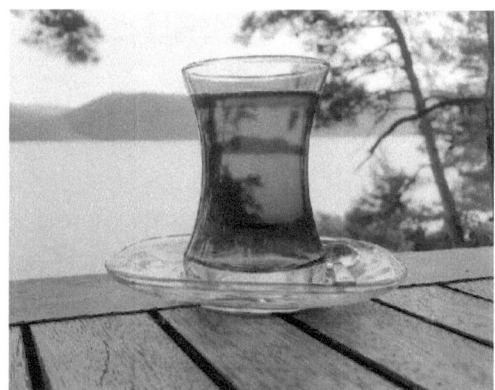

With Ayurvedic origins, spiced tea has been used for generations to help deal with colds. To make spiced tea, here's what you can do:

1. First, make sure to dry roast ¼ cup of coriander seeds together with half a teaspoon each of fennel and cumin seeds, and ¼ tsp. of fenugreek seeds.
2. Then, boil 1 cup of water and add 1 ½ tsp. of the spice powder that you have just made with ½ tsp. of rock candy.
3. Simmer for 3 to 4 minutes.
4. Add 2 tbsp. milk and then boil before straining.

Now, sip the tea while it's still hot, and to try to drink it daily, if you can.

2. <u>Honey</u>

The high enzyme content in honey makes it one of the best remedies for colds. It also has some antibacterial and antiviral properties which aid in immune function.

What you can do is mix 2 tsp. of honey with 1 tsp. of lemon juice. Take this mixture every 2 hours to lessen your symptoms. The remedies in the first chapter for colds can also be utilized for colds.

3. <u>Garlic</u>

Garlic has amazing antibacterial properties and can open up respiratory passages, thereby relieving congestion. Scientifically, there are mixed evidences on whether it really does help with relieving colds. Some suggests that it lessens the severity of the symptoms, but since there is very few research of this nature was conducted, it hasn't been studied thoroughly to a point that proves its efficacy. Regardless, the use of garlic for colds is still going strong.

Preparation:
1. Mix ½ crushed garlic clove with 1 tsp. honey, 2 tsp. lemon juice, and ½ tsp. chili powder or cayenne pepper. Make sure to use it daily until you see the symptoms subsiding.
2. Add garlic oil to your food or drinks, or eat raw garlic, if you can.
3. Boil 4 to 5 garlic cloves with a teaspoon of honey, and drink it at least 2 to 3 times a day.

4. <u>Lemon Essential Oil</u>

Lemon is not only calming, it's also a great anti-viral and antibacterial agent that prevents and helps relieve the symptoms of colds.

You can make a cold remedy this way:

1. Grate the lemon in a bowl.
2. Next, fill up a glass bottle with the grated lemon zest then add some olive oil in the bottle.
3. Place the bottle in a sunny place, preferably a windowsill then let it sit for around 2 weeks, making sure to stir occasionally.

4. After 2 weeks, pour the oil in another clean glass bottle and keep it covered. Store and use as needed.

To use, just dilute with equal parts water and oil, and apply 2 to 4 drops to your throat, wrist, or temples. You may also have it diffused around the house, as well.

Precautions:

Before using any form of essential oils and home remedies, make sure you've tested for allergies. Avoid sun exposure for 12 hours when applying the oil on the skin.

Check your maintenance medication for drug interactions to make sure that there won't be any adverse reaction when using home remedies.

Home Interventions

Salt Water Rinse or Saline Spray

To break up congestion in your nose from mucus build up, try mixing 3 tbsp. of iodide-free salt together with a teaspoon of baking soda. Then, add a teaspoon of the said mixture to 8 oz. of distilled or lukewarm water, and squirt it to your nose with the use of a bulb syringe. Make sure to lean forward while administering the solution so the excess water will drip. Lightly sniff the solution to keep some of it in the nasal cavity. Be careful not to sniff too hard since it can cause irritation when it gets to the back of the throat.

Keep this mixture in an airtight container when not in use.

Breathe Some Steam in

A stuffy nose can be decongested by holding your head over a pot of steaming water, but you have to be extremely careful so that the heat would not burn your nose. Make sure not to stand too close to the water, and keep a safe distance where you can inhale the steam without causing discomfort.

You can also try putting a humidifier in your bedroom, or taking a hot shower with the shower door closed.

Place an Extra Pillow under Your Head

When you elevate yourself while sleeping, the flow of air in your body becomes better. The main reason behind this is that sinus drainage is more continuous in this position which avoids clogging in the sinus cavities. This allows you to breathe easier and prevents the possibility of waking up in the middle of the night and unable to breathe.

MARY CONRAD

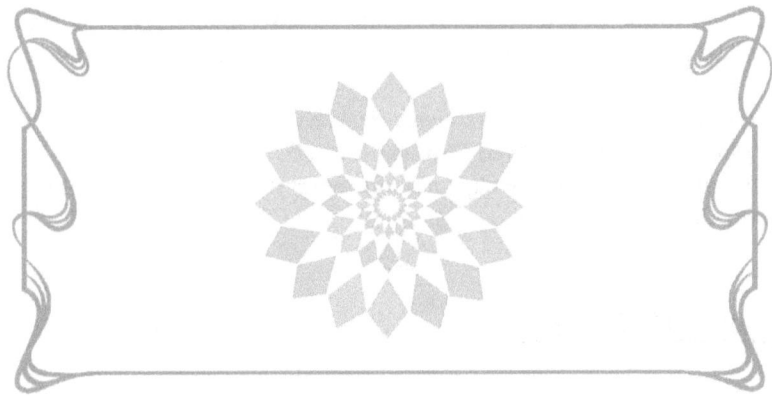

Chapter 6

Sore Throat

Sore throat is a pain or discomfort in the throat, which may include itchiness. The primary manifestation of sore throat is pain on swallowing. Other symptoms include:

- Raw or extreme dryness of the throat,
- Hoarseness
- Inflamed lymph glands or tonsils

Common Causes:

There are different causes for sore throat. It can be bacterial, viral and even environmental.

Viral infections are the most common cause for sore throat. It's usually present when a person has the flu or a cold. Less common viral causes for sore throat include: mononucleosis, measles, chicken pox and croup.

Bacterial infections can also lead to sore throat. Strep throat, which is caused by Streptococcus pyogenes, often cause mild inflammation in the throat and pain. Other conditions include: diphtheria and whooping cough.

Environmental causes for sore throat includes: mold allergies, dry air, excessive talking (such as during lectures) and smoking or exposure to smoke. These are actually quite common as well, since not everything in our environment can be controlled.

Natural Remedies

1. Hot Toddy

A hot toddy is a beverage that soothes your throat, and helps you feel lighter. It's also best to drink this as recommended when you are under the weather. From a scientific standpoint, this drink actually does help with relieving colds and sore throat. The alcohol in whiskey helps in killing off the microorganisms that caused the infection. It's also a vasodilator, which can help decongest the mucus membranes.

For this, you'll need a teaspoon of lemon juice, 4 oz. hot water, 1 tbsp. of honey (or to taste), 1 tsp. lemon juice and 1 oz. of bourbon. Here's what you have to do:

1. Put honey in a mug.
2. Pour some hot water in, and then add lemon juice and bourbon. Make sure to stir well. Enjoy a glass an

2. Slippery Elm

Slippery Elm is a plant that has been studied for years, and has been proven to be a traditional remedy for sore throat. It contains mucilage, a component in the leaves which turns into a gel when mixed with water. This substance stimulates the production of mucus in the linings of the gastrointestinal tract. It helps coat and protect it from conditions such as ulcers and hyperacidity.

You can make you own remedy using the bark. You can manually crush the bark using a mortar and pestle or a food processor. Once its crushed, mix it with water or pour boiling water over the bark. Stir, and then drink what you have mixed. You can take this three times daily for maximum benefits.

Precautions:

There are no major side effects for the intake of this herb. It has a protective effect on the stomach lining by coating it, which in turn delays the absorption of other supplements or herbs. It is advisable to take other supplements two hours after drinking slippery elm to avoid any issues.

For pregnant and nursing women, avoid taking this unless indicated by a health care professional or herbalist. The components of the bark of this herb is said to cause miscarriages.

3.   Marshmallow Root

This has been used in Europe and North America for a couple of centuries now because it has been proven to soothe irritated mucus membranes. It also contains mucilage and has similar properties to slippery elm.

What you can do here is just mix a cup of boiling water with 1 tbsp. of dried marshmallow root, and then put a tablespoon of this root mixture in a mug before pouring boiling water. Steep for at least 30 to 60 minutes, with lid covered, strain, and drink.

Precautions:

Marshmallow is generally considered safe with little side effects. Some studies suggest that it may lower blood sugar levels, so for those who have diabetes, you need to check with your health care provider or naturopathic doctor prior to usage. Pregnant and nursing women also need to check with their naturopathic doctor prior to intake.

4.   Salt water

According to the *University of Puget Sound,* by simply gargling with salted warm water, you'd get to break secretions in your throat that cause sore throat. It kills bacteria, as well.

Just add ½ tsp. of salt to a glass of warm water, gargle it, and see the effects.

5. <u>Garlic</u>

Again, garlic has some antibacterial and anti-viral properties that help relieve sore throat. It contains the compound allicin—which is attributed for its bactericidal effect. According to a study, the allicin in garlic was effective in both Gram positive and Gram negative bacteria.

For this remedy, just do the following:

1. Place a piece of garlic in each of your cheeks.
2. Then, suck on those garlic pieces like you would a cough drop.
3. Now, crush your teeth against it so the allicin could be released. Make sure to do this daily for it to work better.

6. **Apple Cider Vinegar**

Apple Cider Vinegar (ACV) is mostly used for both health and home for its various health benefits. Due to its high levels of acidity, it is able to kill bacteria right away. Most bacteria can't survive in an acidic environment which explains why this remedy is quite effective.

For your sore throat remedy, you'll need a cup of warm water, 1 tbsp. honey, and 1 tbsp. ACV. Now, follow the instructions below:

1. In warm water, mix ACV and honey together and make sure to drink while it's still warm.
2. Or, you can also mix 2 tbsp. of ACV with a cup of warm water and use it for gargling at least once a day.

Precautions:

If you have tooth problems avoid gargling ACV, since it can cause erosion of the tooth enamel.

7. **Drink Cayenne Pepper Tea**

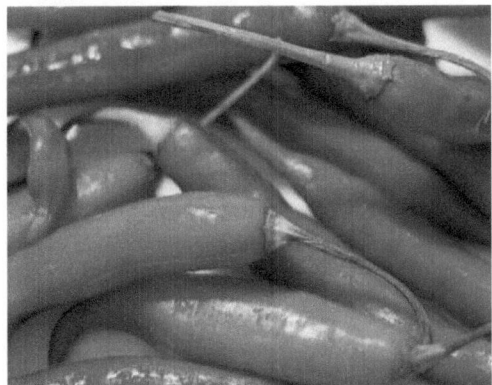

Cayenne contains capsaicin. Now, you may be familiar with this because it aids in weight loss, but another great thing about it is that it actually relieves pain, and also kills bacteria in the mouth—which often causes sore throat. It also prevents pain signals from being transmitted to the brain, which can give some relief from pain.

Prepare a tsp. of honey, 1 cup of boiling water, and ½ tsp. of cayenne powder. Then, simply follow the instructions below:

1. Prepare a cup of hot water, and add ½ tsp. of cayenne powder.
2. Pour the honey and stir until the it dissolves into the mixture. Drink it all throughout your day.
3. Stir frequently before drinking. You can adjust the ratios of cayenne to ¼ or less if you're sensitive to spices.

Precautions:

Those who have latex allergy or food allergies with kiwis, bananas, chestnuts and avocados may also be allergic to cayenne.

Home Intervention

Give your throat a break. Try and avoid instances where you'll be forced to shout and cause more stress and pain on your throat. Try to avoid cold beverages which can aggravate the condition.

When to seek medical attention:

Normally, sore throat resolves on its own, but there are cases where you may need to see a doctor. When you experience symptoms for about a week or more and it's accompanied by any of these symptoms:

- Difficulty in breathing
- High fever at 101 °F
- Blood in the mucus
- Rashes
- Difficulty in swallowing
- Joint pain and swelling
- Ear ache
- Lump in your throat

Chapter 7

Bug Bites

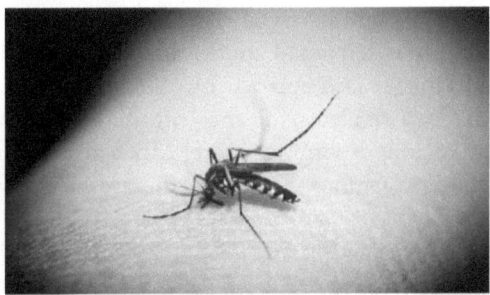

Bug bites are usually minor and only lasts for a day or two. While some insects bite intentionally, there are also those who only bite when provoked or when you accidentally stumble on their nest.

Bug bites that are from mosquitoes, bed bugs, ticks and lice are often intentional whereas those from spiders, fire ants, bees and hornets are usually to protect their territory. The latter needs to be avoided as much as possible. Diseases can be transmitted through these bites, so it's always a good idea to prevent being bitten.

Minor bug bites will have the following manifestations:

- Swelling
- Itchiness
- Redness
- Heat around the affected area
- Occasionally some bites can lead to numbness in the area

Natural Remedies

1. **Vinegar**

A simple way of cleaning the bite area is by using vinegar. Again, because of high levels of acid, vinegar easily fights bacteria and kills the pathogens which may invade the affected area.

It's best to use ACV, but any type of vinegar you have on hand will be fine. Since bug bites are often small and localized you can just soak a cotton ball with undiluted vinegar and apply it on the area. Wait until the swelling and itching subsides before removing the cotton. Another way to treat bites using vinegar is by making a vinegar paste: Mix a teaspoon of vinegar with flour or cornstarch. You can apply this on the area for a few minutes until relief is felt.

2. **Tea Tree Oil**

If you hate mosquitoes and other kinds of insects, then Tea Tree Oil is your friend. If you use it on the skin, it can act as an insect repellant that has been proven to be truly effective

When mosquitoes bite, they release anticoagulants into the body so they can efficiently take the blood. The body responds by releasing histamine which triggers the inflammatory process. This explains why the area becomes itchy and swollen. Tea tree oil helps by reducing the inflammation caused by histamine.

To make tea tree oil, just follow these instructions:

1. Put some tea tree leaves in a pot. Pour enough water to cover the leaves. Take a vegetable steamer and place it over the pot of tea tree leaves and water. Place a glass measuring cup in the vegetable steamer. When covering the pot and steamer, flip it so the lid handle is directly above the cup.
2. Boil the leaves on high heat. Once the leaves start to boil and leaves are steaming, add a few ice cubes. This will help by increasing the rate of condensation. Allow the condensation to drip and collect inside the measuring cup.
3. Turn off the burner once all the ice has melted then take off the lid and pour ice down the sink.
4. Close the stopcock of the separatory funnel and pour in the contents of the measuring cup. Close the top opening of the funnel. Shake the mixture thoroughly.
5. Invert the funnel and open the top lid so pressure could be released and then wait for the oil to float above the water. Put the glass in the stockpot and drain the water. Repeat process with the remaining leaves.
6. Place contents in a jar and store in a cool, dry place. Use whenever necessary.

Once you have the oil, you can apply a drop of it on the bite area. You'll notice a difference around 10 minutes after the application.

Precautions:

Use cautiously when pregnant and nursing. May cause slight hormonal changes when applied in the chest area so avoid applying the oil on that area, especially for pre-pubescent and pubescent boys.

Perform a skin test by applying a diluted form of the oil to a patch of skin. If there's any signs of redness and inflammation within 24 hours, avoid using the oil. Do not ingest the oil unless you have a health care provider and professional who is trained on the use of essential oils.

3. Tea Bags

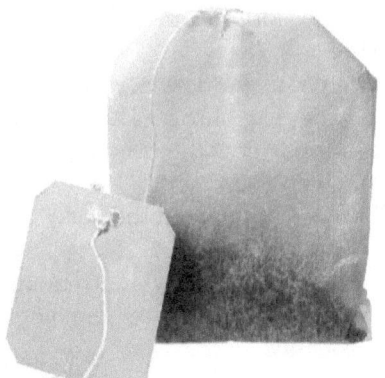

Get some cool tea bags and place them where you have been bitten. The tea bag is believed to draw out the fluid from a bite as well reduce both swelling and itching! The anti-inflammatory properties of tea have some effect on the skin making it quite effective.

4. Ice

Ice can help by reducing swelling and numbing the nerves in the area. It can also help release the body's natural anti-histamine—which means that not only will you be able to end the pain of bug bites, it will also reduce the urge to scratch the itch.

Try making an ice pack and place it on the bite/sting for a good 15 minutes. Do this at intervals if the swelling is severe. Be careful not to leave it on your skin for too long, and make sure not to sleep with it, as well.

5. Basil

While it's one of the favorite spices of many, basil actually contains camphor—a compound that creates a cooling sensation! It is also an effective insect repellant and can penetrate into the skin to help relieve itching. There's little scientific studies which prove the effectiveness of this remedy, but it is generally considered safe to use.

What you can do is crush a couple leaves of basil and apply it directly to where the bites and bumps are. Observe closely for any signs of allergies.

6. Mix Water and Milk

You need to mix equal parts of water and skim milk. Dip an old t-shirt or a thin piece of cloth in the mixture, and then just dab it on your skin.

The protein contained in milk is said to be responsible for this healing effect on the skin.

7. Tape or cellophane

If you have been bitten by a puss caterpillar, you could ease the pain by placing tape or cellophane over the broken-off caterpillar spines to take them out. You could also opt to use facial peel—if you have some. Just place them on the affected areas, to remove the spines and proceed with any of the natural remedies above to help with the pain and any swelling.

Home Interventions

For bee stings, the stinger needs to removed. If the venom sack is still attached, it needs to be extracted carefully without too much contact with the affected area. The main reason for this is to avoid the venom from spreading further into the skin. You can scrape the area using your fingernails or a hard card to gently dislodge it.

Basic Home Treatment for Minor Bites/Stings:

- Gently wash the affected area with soap and water.
- Avoid scratching the area which can aggravate the itchiness and lead to infections.
- Apply cold compress to relieve the swelling.

When going on hikes and relishing the great outdoors, it's always a great idea to take preventive measures to avoid a bad experience such as being bitten by ticks or being a buffet for mosquitoes. Here are a few tips to avoid bites and stings:

- Dress well enough to cover exposed areas such as arms, legs and neck.
- Wear a hat
- Avoid bright colors and instead go for neutrals.
- Avoid using scented lotion or perfumes.
- Store food in airtight containers.
- Keep insect repellents handy
- You can also use citronella candles to keep the bugs away.

When to seek medical assistance:

Bites are often localized but for those who have allergies, it might cause a systemic reaction. Here are a few warning signs to keep in mind.

- Difficulty in breathing
- Muscle spasms or seizures
- Fever
- Vomiting

- Palpitations
- Loss of consciousness
- Severe swelling in the lips or face

Once there are signs of severe allergic reaction, it is best to seek medical assistance immediately.

MARY CONRAD

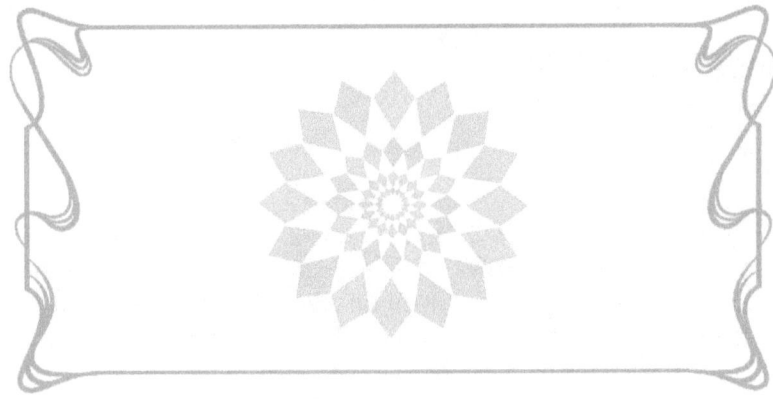

Chapter 8

Bruises

A bruise is a discoloration of the skin which usually starts off as a red spot then blue and purple. This is caused by injury such us bumping into objects and happens when capillaries burst underneath the skin. The blood then leaks into the tissues and muscles and stops just underneath the skin.

There are instances where bruising is more common such as when taking blood thinners, which makes one bleed easily. The elderly also bruise easily due to their skin being thinner.

Bruises often take about two weeks to disappear completely, and doesn't need much attention.

Natural Remedies

1. Pineapples

Bromelain in pineapple is a fibrolytic agent, which helps in reducing the formation of clots. It stimulates the conversion of plasminogen to plasmin, which increases the breakdown of fibrin. Basically, this enzyme delays the clotting time as well as helps breakdown clots that have been formed.

Drinking pineapple juice or eating pineapples don't give enough bromelain to reduce bruises. It's best to use supplements to make it more effective. You can take 250 mg of bromelain two to three times daily until the bruises look better.

For those of you who have access to organic pineapples, you can actually make bromelain-rich tea out of the pineapple skins and leftover leaves. The concentration of the enzymes is actually higher in the leaves and skin compared to the fruit itself. Here is how you can prepare pineapple leaf tea:

Ingredients:
- Pineapple leaves or skin (whichever you have handy)
- Stevia or honey
- One liter of water

Directions:
1. Wash the pineapple skins and leaves thoroughly. Cut into small pieces.
2. Add the leaves into a pot with one liter of water.
3. Cover and let it boil in low heat for 20 minutes.
4. Let it cool for 5 minutes and sweeten.

Apply Poultices

There are different kinds of poultices you can use for bruises, and these are the following:

1. **Cabbage**: Get white cabbage leaves and wash them. Break into veins or ridges and place where you have been bruised.

2. **Oatmeal**: Cook some oatmeal. Let it sit for a few minutes. Test it on the skin if the warmth is tolerable. After which, directly apply it to where you have been bruised to decrease inflammation.

3. **Mustard**: For bruised and inflamed ankles and joints, get some crushed mustard seeds and add to your foot bath. You can also crush some of the seeds and add some honey. Apply it on the affected area to help hasten healing. It works by helping breakdown the clots under the skin. It also prevents congestion from happening in most parts of your body. Use it with olive oil for better effects, as well.

4. **Marjoram**: The leaves of this plant is a known for its antioxidant and anti-inflammatory properties. It can be used for wound healing, bruises and other gastrointestinal issues. Mix it with equal parts of flaxseed in a pot of boiling water. Let the mixture cool until warm but not scalding. Use clean cloth to dip into the mixture, and then apply it to the bruised area. This also works for sprains, earaches, and toothaches, as well.

5. **Witch Hazel:** It works by contracting the underlying tissues and blood vessels, which stops further bruising and helps it heal faster. Get some witch hazel tincture and use absorbent cotton to help you apply it on the affected area.

6. **Vinegar:** Warm a thin cloth by ironing or steaming. Dip the thin cloth into a bowl of vinegar and wring it out. Once it's wrung, fold it into the bruised area and let it stay there for a little while. The vinegar increases the circulation in the area and helps breakdown the clots.

7. **Sage:** Place some cool sage on abrasions that are raw, cover with cloth, and have it enclosed for an hour or two. It works by contracting the surrounding tissues which limits the spread of

the bruise.

8. **Potato:** Grate raw potato and apply it on the bruised area. Its alkaline juices serve as an antiseptic.

9. **Onion:** Roast some onions and place it in a pack—like an ice pack. Then, simply apply what you have made to the bruised or wounded area. It serves and an analgesic and anti-inflammatory, which aids in healing.

Precautions:

Perform a skin test for allergies prior to using these poultices. Apply a small amount of the poultice in a patch of skin and observe between 30 minutes to 24 hours. If there are signs of irritation, redness and inflammation. It wouldn't be a good idea to use it.

2. <u>Parsley</u>

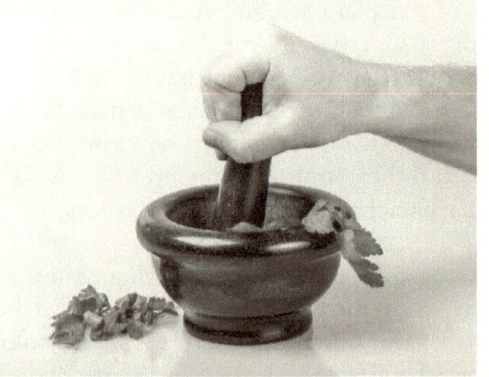

Studies have shown that parsley is an effective anti-inflammatory agent, which can aid in reducing bruises. A surprising fact about this herb is that it's also has hepatoprotective properties against several liver toxins that lead to inflammation.

For bruises, simply cut up fresh parsley and apply it on the bruised area. Bind it with elastic bandage to secure and keep it in place. Continue application until the bruise is lessened.

Home Interventions

Cold Compress

For the first 24 hours after getting a bruise, apply ice on the area to reduce inflammation and pain. Once ice is applied, the surrounding blood vessels will constrict which reduces the possibility of further bruising in the area. The cold will also numb the nerve endings which will temporarily ease the pain.

Let the compress stay for 15 minutes at a time for between 3-4 hours' interval depending on the size and severity of the injury.

Hot Compress

This one's a classic.

Simply get a cloth or towel and dip it into hot water. Once it's warm and the heat is tolerable, place it over the bruised area. This is best done after 24 hours. The heat will promote healing as well as breakdown the clots formed under the skin. It is then mobilized for excretion from the system but may take a while to take effect.

The time length and frequency is similar with the cold compress. The rationale behind this is that the compress is only effective for 15 minutes of contact. After that time frame, it is no longer beneficial and can cause tissue damage.

When to seek medical assistance:

There are a few things to look for that may indicate a more serious condition. In situations where you have any of the signs listed below, medical assistance may be required:

- When there no reason for the bruising but it's there. This is especially true for those who are taking blood thinners.
- The bruise is not healing.
- When there is pain and swelling with the bruise (might be a sprain or fracture).

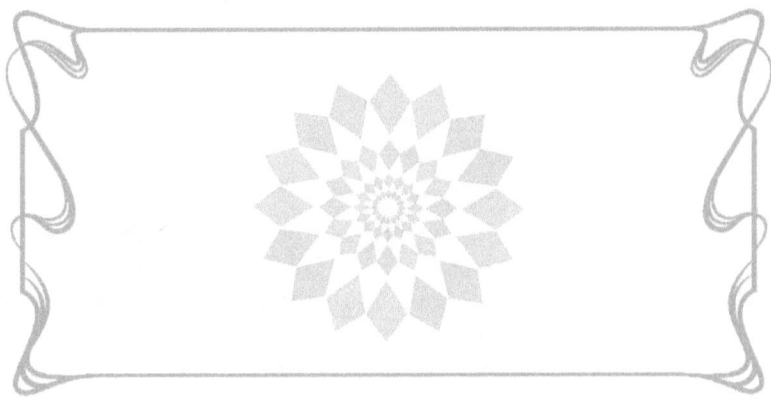

Chapter 9

Sprain and Strain

A sprain is an injury where the ligaments, which holds the joints in place, gets torn off either partially or completely. This usually occurs in knees and ankles since these often bear our weight and can easily be twisted. The severity of the sprain often depends on the pain and swelling, which are the initial signs of the injury. It can range from mild to severe depending on whether or not weight can be placed on the affected area.

A strain is an injury to the tendons or muscles such as tearing due to being stretched to its limits then shortened or contracted too quickly. This can cause the muscle to twist and cause tears. This is a common injury of the lower back and hamstring muscles of the leg.

Symptoms include:
- Pain in the affected area
- Swelling and redness
- Muscle spasm as well as weakness

Natural Remedies

1. Garlic

The organosulphur compounds in garlic help in halting the inflammatory response. In several primary studies, it has been proven that garlic also halts the development of adipose tissues, which have been linked as a potential cause for increased inflammatory response in the body as well as obesity. For sprains, it helps ease the swelling.

Preparation:

1. Mix a tablespoon of garlic juice with 2 tbsp. of warm coconut oil.
2. Use the solution on the affected area by having it rubbed there and leave it for at least 30 minutes before washing. Do this 3 to 4 times a day until the sprain has healed.
3. Or, you can also mix a teaspoon of garlic with almond oil. Use it to massage the sprained area with for at least 2 to 3 times each day, and make sure to repeat until you have fully recovered. This also works for rheumatism and arthritis.

2. Arnica

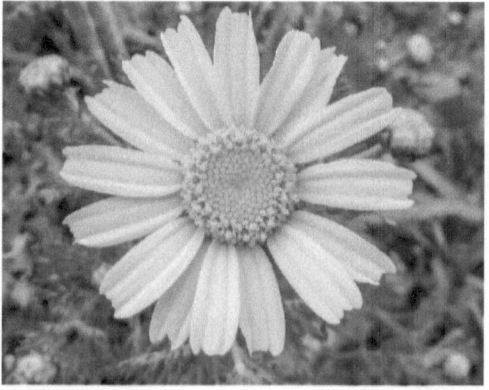

Arnica is a natural anti-inflammatory agent that reduces swelling, prevents more bruising, and improves circulation of blood and oxygen to make healing easier.

Here's what you can do:

1. Use arnica ointment or balm and use it for compression twice or thrice a day.
2. Apply arnica on the affected area and massage the said area.

Enclose it with wrap and leave it on for 5 to 6 hours to induce healing.

Precautions:

This herb is usually safe for topical applications but may lead to skin irritation with prolonged use. It is not advisable to use on open wounds since it can cause more pain in the area. Ingesting arnica should be monitored by a homeopathic doctor or herbalist since there are side effects such as dizziness, tremors and heart irregularities.

3. <u>Onions</u>

Onions belong to the same family as garlic — Allium, which explains it's anti-inflammatory properties.

Here's how you can prepare this remedy:

1. First, chop an onion into small pieces, and place it into a muslin cloth. Tie the cloth and put it on the affected area for at least 2 hours. Keep using until swelling subsides or relief is felt.
2. Alternatively, refrigerate chopped onions for two hours and mix with salt. Place on the swollen part of the body and wrap with elastic bandage. Apply every 2 days until you are healed.

4. <u>Castor Oil</u>

This oil is an old Japanese remedy, which aids in improving gastrointestinal issues and inflammatory conditions. Although this oil is hardly used for internal use in this day and age, it is still widely used for topical applications.

Preparation:

1. Make a pad by folding a piece of cloth several times.
2. Now, get the pad and dip it into castor oil.
3. Get a bottle of hot water and place it on the castor pack for at least 30 minutes.
4. Elevate your sprained ankle for a couple of minutes and then lightly massage the rest of the oil on your skin.
5. Repeat this treatment for at least 2 to 3 times in a matter of 2 days.

Precautions:

For pregnant and lactating women, intake of the oil should be discussed with a health care professional such as naturopathic doctor. Those who have gastrointestinal issues should avoid taking the oil without consent from a physician.

Home Interventions

For minor sprains and strains, it can easily be treated at home. Initially, you can refer to the acronym **RICE (Rest, Ice, Compression and Elevation)** as a first line of treatment.

Rest: Once injury is sustained, the person must rest the affected area on a flat surface. It may be advised to keep the area immobilized for the first 48 hours after sustaining the injury. You can either use a splint or crutches to avoid putting weight on the injured ankle or knee. After the 48-hour mark, try putting some weight on the area to check if it's not too painful. A bit of light movement in the area can help with circulation and healing.

Ice: Apply a pack of ice on the area to help with the pain and reduce the swelling. Keep the pack on the are for about 15-20 minutes for about 4 to 8 times a day for the first 2 days. This is to reduce the swelling in the area. Please note that the ice pack shouldn't be left on the area for longer than 20 minutes since it may lead to more tissue damage.

Compression: Compression can help support the affected area. You can use an elastic bandage or neoprene sleeves if you prefer.

Elevation: This can help reduce the swelling in the injured joint.

When to seek medical attention:

There's always a possibility of a more serious issue when dealing with injury in the muscles and tendons. If you have any of the signs and symptoms indicated below, it is imperative to get medical assistance:
- Repeated injury in the same area
- Inability to place weight on the affected knee or ankle.
- Severe and debilitating pain
- Unable to move the joint
- Numbness in the area
- Appearance of red striations from the affected joint which can indicate infection

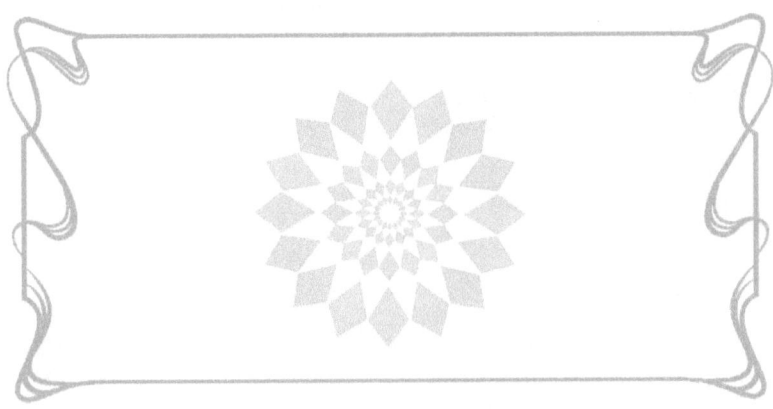

Chapter 10

Fever

Fever is often a sign of infection. It's more of a symptom rather than an illness on its own. Think of fever as a warning signal from our body that alerts us when foreign bodies enter our system. The reason why the body heats up is to create a conducive environment for our antibodies to fight and at the same time increase the production of these cells as needed.

For infants, there may not be any visible signs of temperature elevation but it could be backwards. They could instead have a lower body temperature than normal. This also needs medical attention. Warning signs for infants include: lethargy, irritability and loss of appetite. Also look for signs of dehydration such as sunken fontanels and poor skin turgor.

For toddlers, any fever that persists for more than 24 hours at 102 °F, may need medical attention. This is best to check for potential infections rather than have regrets later on, especially if the fever is accompanied by vomiting, diarrhea and loss of appetite. If the toddler is playing normally and able to respond well then it may not be any cause for concern.

For adults, if your fever is accompanied by other discomforts such as severe pain, seizures, confusion and other unexplained symptoms then it is best to get medical help. Three days of persistent fever with temperatures at

103 °F to 106 °F require medical attention.

Fever may be accompanied by:
- Shivering
- Muscle aches
- Sweating
- Loss of appetite
- Fatigue

A body temperature of over 103 °F can manifest:
- Confusion
- Convulsion
- Dehydration
- Irritability
- Hallucinations

Note: This requires immediate medical attention.

Natural Remedies

1. Raisin Juice

The use of raisin juice, watered down wine and grapes for fever and inflammation has deep roots in the Jewish culture. In recent studies, it has been proven that grapes and its extracts have many health benefits. It's a great antioxidant and can help boost the immune function. Here's what you can do:

1. Soak some raisins—at least 25 to 30 of them—in ½ cup water until soft, or for a good 30 minutes.
2. Now, crush those raisins with the water. Strain the juice.
3. Use ½ lime juice with it, and drink the juice twice a day until your fever has subsided.

2. Apple Cider Vinegar

Vinegar has antibacterial properties, which is mainly due to acetic acid. It penetrates the bacterial cell membrane which kills off the pathogen. This may be the reason why this remedy works in lowering body temperature. It can actually penetrate the skin, which explains its systemic effects.

What you can do is this:

1. *ACV Bath Soak*: Mix ½ cup of vinegar with lukewarm bath water. Soak in the said bath for 5 to 10 minutes.
2. *ACV Wash*: Get a clean washcloth and soak it with 2 parts water and one part of apple cider vinegar (ACV). Wring the cloth out and place it on your tummy and forehead. Wrap on the soles of your feet, as well, if you can, and repeat until your fever has gone down.
3. *ACV Tonic*: Mix it with honey and drink twice or thrice a day.

Precautions:

Make sure that ACV is heavily diluted since it may cause damage to the enamel and mouth. Wash out the mouth after drinking ACV to ensure that it is washed out.

3. Make Yourself Some Tea

Some teas could alleviate the pain or discomfort that you might feel as you lie in bed. Here are certain teas that you could make—and drink!

1. **Lavender.** Fever, and tension headaches can be lessened with the help of Lavender Tea. Lavender relieves stress, and could also help one sleep better—so you definitely have to drink it as much as you can. Lavender also works against anxiety and nervous exhaustion. Aside from that, it also regulates the digestive process—so with its help, you can be holistically healthy!

   It may not directly address the fever but it does have antibacterial properties which can boost the immune function. You can make lavender tea by using lavender flowers. Get three tablespoons of dried or fresh flowers. Add it to two cups of boiling water. Let it simmer for 5-10 minutes. Once it has cooled, add a sweetener of your choice and a lemon wedge for flavor.

   Precautions:

   Always make sure to test for allergies before using the oil for both diffusion and topical applications. For pregnant and nursing women, avoid using lavender.

2. **Lemon Verbana.** This is another tea that's perfect for those with fever. It also combats nausea that's often brought on by an stomach. This is an old folk remedy for fever, but has proven to be effective for Gram positive bacteria. It also has some antifungal properties.

3. **Ginseng.** Ginseng immediately clears out stress and mental exhaustion. Just after drinking a cup, you'd already feel lighter, and you'd feel at peace. According to the University of Maryland Medical Center, this root may help boost the immune function, which shortens the duration of fever, colds and flu. Ginseng could also help you sleep better, so do drink a cup during bed time.

   Precautions:

   • Ginseng is not advisable to take for long periods without consulting a professional who knows how to properly dose it for long term use. This may also increase the risk of developing side effects.

- Try not to take ginseng with caffeine since it can increase feelings of nervousness as well as affect the sleeping patterns.
- This root needs to be taken with food since it can affect the blood sugar levels.
- Those with autoimmune disorders should steer clear of this remedy since it has a potential to aggravate the immune response.
- Pregnant and nursing women are not advised to take any supplements containing ginger. The same is true for those who are breast cancer survivors.
- Those with high blood pressure require medical supervision when taking ginseng

4. **Catnip.** This herb is commonly used to relieve stress and anxiety as well as promote quality sleep. When made into a tea, it can induce perspiration which makes it effective when treating fever. It helps cool off the body as well as relax and relieve discomfort from other conditions such as colds and flu. It's also effective for nervousness and hyperactivity

You can make your own tea by boiling one cup of water. Once boiled, transfer it on a cup. Add one teaspoon of dried catnip or three fresh leaves, if you have any. Let it steep for 20 minutes. Strain the mixture, and add a sweetener of choice once the drink cools.

Precautions:

High doses can cause extreme drowsiness. It would be a great idea to talk to a professional prior to usage.

3. <u>Garlic Once Again</u>

It is believed that garlic can cause the body to perspire, which lowers the body temperature. What you can do is this:

1. Mix ½ crushed garlic clove with 1 tsp. honey, 2 tsp. lemon juice, and ½ tsp. chili powder or cayenne pepper. Make sure to use it daily until you see that symptoms subsiding.

2. Add garlic oil to your food or drinks, or eat raw garlic, if you can.
3. Boil 4 to 5 garlic cloves with a teaspoon of honey, and drink it at least 2 to 3 times a day.
4. Place a piece of garlic in each of your cheeks.
5. Then, suck on those garlic pieces like you would a cough drop.
6. Now, crush your teeth against it so the allicin could be released. Make sure to do this daily for it to work better.

4. <u>Ginger</u>

Ginger is another natural anti-viral and antibacterial agent, which means that it's quite helpful when it comes to helping you heal from varied types of infections. What you can do is this:

1. Put 2 tbsp. of ginger powder in a tub filled with warm water. Get in the tub and soak in the water for a good 10 minutes, and then go to sleep after patting your body dry. Use a blanket to cover yourself with completely.
2. Add a teaspoon of freshly grated ginger with boiling water. Steep for a few minutes, and drink 3 to 4 times a day.
3. Mix ginger juice with honey and lemon juice and drink 3 to 4 times a day—or until your fever is gone.

5. <u>Egg Whites</u>

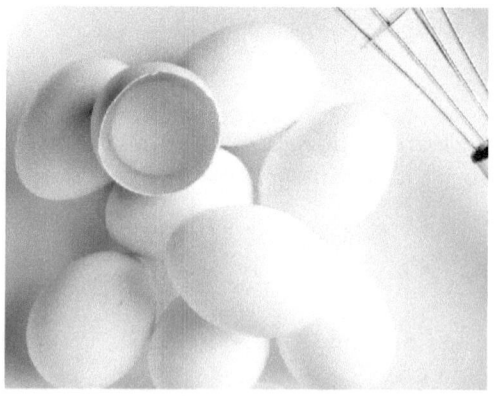

There are no studies to support this remedy, but it is believed that egg whites draw the heat from the head to the feet. It's an effective and fast remedy when you are experiencing a high fever. Several people who have tried this swears to its effectiveness, since it is very non-invasive it's still a good home cure to try out. This is how you prepare the remedy:

1. Break an egg or two and have the yolk separated.
2. Now, work on the egg white by beating it for at least a minute.

3. Soak a thin cloth on the egg white.
4. Place the cloth on the soles of your feet, and once they're dry, replace them with new ones.
5. Repeat until your fever has alleviated.

Home Interventions

A tepid sponge bath can go a long way in increasing comfort and cooling the skin.

1. Take a medium-sized basin or bowl.
2. Fill it with cool water, making sure it's not too hot or too cold.
3. Soak a bath sponge or small towel. Wring out the excess moisture.
4. Wash the exposed skin.
5. Continue doing the bath until the fever breaks.

MARY CONRAD

Chapter 11

Minor Allergies

An allergic reaction is a condition wherein the body reacts to certain substances, which usually isn't threat to health. This is quite common in children and adults alike. The immune system reacts to these substances by activating tear ducts (watery eyes), sneezing fits, coughing, breakout of hives or rashes. Most of these reactions are easily managed at home by using home remedies or over-the-counter medication such as antihistamines and decongestants.

In rare cases a severe allergic reaction (anaphylaxis) can occur. This is marked by:

- Swelling of the airways
- Difficulty of breathing
- Lightheadedness
- Confusion

Note: Anaphylaxis is a life threatening condition and requires immediate medical attention. For those who have known severe allergies, ask your physician to supply you with information on obtaining an EpiPen (epinephrine) for emergency situations.

Natural Remedies

1.   Saline Rinse and Neti Pot

Place a sterile saline solution inside the neti pot, and you'll be able to flush out allergens and other forms of irritations—while clearing your airways, too.

You can use a pre-made rinse, or dissolve sea or Himalayan salt with water. Pour it into the pot and into your nostril, and let it be drained out.

2.   ACV

According to naturopaths, ACV works against seasonal allergies by balancing the gut. It contains enzymes, which is beneficial for gut health. Once the gut is clean, it is believed to result into less instances of flare ups from allergies. For this, you'll need a cup of warm water, 1 tbsp. honey, and 1 tbsp. ACV. Now, follow the instructions below:

1.   In warm water, mix ACV and honey together and make sure to drink while it's still warm.
2.   Or, you can also mix 2 tbsp. of ACV with a cup of warm water and use it for gargling at least once a day!

3.   Nettle Leaf

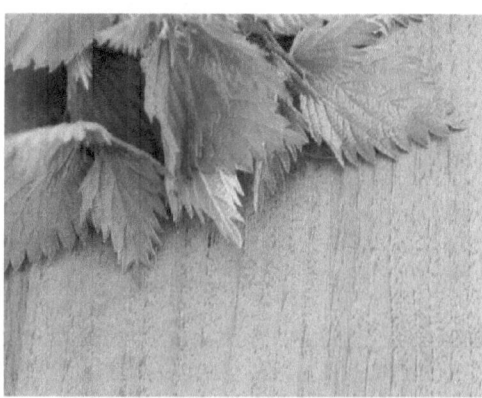

This is a natural anti-histamine so it's certainly a winner for this category and is effective because it really blocks histamine or allergen production in the body. You can mix it with other herbs or use it on its own as a tea or tincture. Just add it to your usual cup of tea, and you're all set! If you can buy nettle leaf capsules, that would help you out as well.

Precautions:

If you're taking any maintenance medication, consult your doctor prior to use.

4. Butterbur

Butterbur works well with nasal allergies. It helps by suppressing the inflammatory process triggered by leukotriene. After five days of treatment, there's a marked difference in the levels of histamine and leukotriene in the body.

It's an effective remedy in pill form but has not yet been proven to be effective for skin allergies.

Precautions:

Before taking butterbur, make sure to acquire one which has no pyrrolizidine alkaloids (PAs), which can cause liver problems. Only those items which are labelled PA-free are safe to use. It's been proven safe to take between 12-16 weeks for adults but children require medical supervision before taking the herb.

Those who are allergic to chrysanthemums, marigolds, ragweed and daises should avoid butterbur.

5. Add Turmeric to Your Meals

Turmeric is known for its anti-inflammatory properties, but research has shown that it also helps in alleviating the discomforts of food allergies. It reduces diarrhea and anaphylactic symptoms, as well as, inhibits the production of cytokines, which are responsible for inflammation.

Home Intervention

Get Appliances with HEPA Filters

Appliances with HEPA Filters help against allergies because they pick up pollen and other allergens swarming around your house. This way, allergy symptoms would be minimized, and air becomes cleaner, as well.

Wear a mask

During months where pollen is floating in the air, wearing a mask is a great way of keeping the sniffles at bay. It'll protect your airways and doesn't cost a small fortune.

Always Change Your Clothes When You Come Home

This way, you can easily let go of bacteria and germs that you may have brought home with you—and it's always best to feel clean, and in "new" clothes, too.

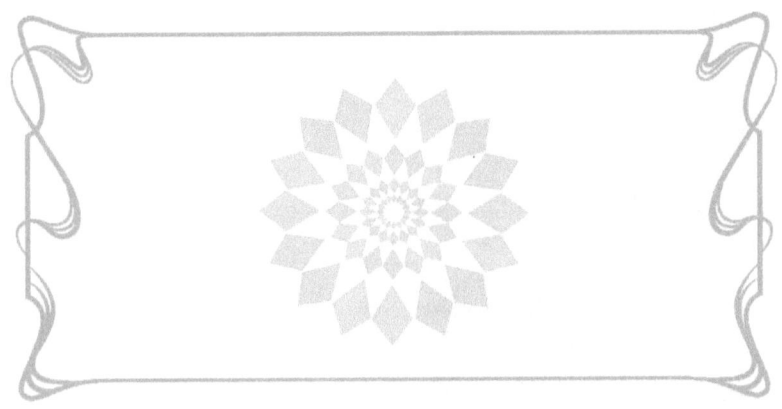

Chapter 12

Dyspepsia

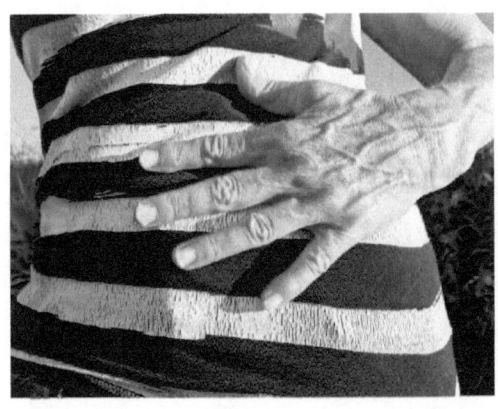

Dyspepsia is a condition wherein there is an abnormal function within the gastrointestinal tract, which leads to symptoms similar to indigestion.

Symptoms include:

- Stomach pain
- Bloating
- Discomfort after eating or early satiety
- Heartburn
- Loss of desire to eat

- Regurgitation
- Excessive burping
- Distended abdomen

For the most part, dyspepsia is often a minor condition with very few cases requiring medical attention. The common causes of this condition are the following:

- Intake of NSAIDs (Non-steroidal Anti-inflammatory Drugs)
- Anxiety and depression
- Lactose intolerance
- Swallowed air
- Inflammatory Bowel Syndrome
- GERD (Gastroesophageal Reflux Disease) or hiatal hernia

Natural Remedies

1. **Chew a Carrot**

Carrots are high in fiber, vitamins and minerals. The fiber in this vegetable aids in cleansing the colon, and keeping the intestinal tract healthy. Several research has been conducted that showed its anti-cancer properties, specifically for those with colon cancer. Further studies need to be conducted, but it has great potential for an alternative treatment for this type of cancer.

It's also an antimicrobial, which help in inhibiting the spread of food borne bacteria and yeast.

You can take raw carrot juice for maximum benefits or even eat steamed ones.

2. **Anise Seeds**

Anise seeds aid in relieving some of the symptoms of dyspepsia such as bloating and gas. It has an antispasmodic effect, which relaxes the intestinal tract relieving any cramping, gas and bloating. It has some antibacterial and antifungal properties as well.

Taking the seeds can also relieve flatulence.

3. Butter Milk

This is another simple—and quite delicious—home cure for dyspepsia. This is an old folk remedy that is said to coat the stomach lining and relaxes the intestinal tract.

What you can do is prepare a glass of buttermilk, and then add cumin or black pepper, and drink it at least twice or thrice a day until your dyspepsia eases out.

4. Tangerine Oil

Meanwhile, Tangerine Essential Oil, which is made out of tangerine rind, is often used as a sedative because of its great calming properties. This oil is also a good source of Vitamin C, which makes it an amazing anti-inflammatory agent and also contains high amounts of potassium and magnesium. It has anti-spasmodic properties, which helps in relieving flatulence and digestive issues.

To make this oil, simply follow the instructions below:

1. Scrape off the peel of the tangerine. It would be helpful to use a citrus zester.
2. Next, fill a glass bottle or jar with the tangerine zest then mix some olive oil inside the jar. Make sure that the tangerine is completely covered in oil.
3. Put the jar somewhere sunny and just leave it be for 2 to 4 weeks but make sure to shake it once or twice daily.
4. Strain the mixture and discard any excess tangerine peels. Store in a cool, dry place and use as needed.

Use by diluting with 50% water and applying to vital points. It can be applied on the stomach for a more direct result.

Precautions:

May lead to sensitivity with continued use. Avoid sunlight for 12 hours when applied in areas which is exposed to the sun.

5. Try Metabolism-Boosting Teas

Sometimes, dyspepsia may be a result of slow metabolism, which can be a direct result of hormonal imbalances, poor food choices and inactivity. For these conditions, you can use metabolism-boosting teas—such as these ones below:

1. **Star Anise Tea.** Star Anise is native to China and has always been known to treat most digestive troubles, especially diarrhea and stomach upset. Steep a whole pod for around 10 minutes in hot water to get maximum effects of the tea. Make sure to strain and sweeten, because drinking it without any other ingredients may make you hate the whole thing as it might be too bitter for your taste.

2. **Porangaba.** Porangaba mostly grows in Brazil and other places in South America, and is known as Brazil's very own weight loss potion. The leaves of the Porangaba plant resemble coffee. In fact, it also contains caffeine, but the amount is just right, and wouldn't bring forth undesirable side effects. The caffeine content is what boosts the metabolism and fat-burning in the body. Porangaba acts as a diuretic that reduces appetite and naturally boosts weight loss. Remember that it's best to drink a tea bag of Porangaba at least 30 minutes before each meal starts.

Precautions:

Avoid using this tea when pregnant and nursing. For those who are taking lithium supplements, consult your physician since this tea helps slow the excretion of lithium in the body. It's also a diuretic.

3. **Oolong.** Oolong is known to enhance metabolism, and is also used to prevent the body from forming more fat than necessary, which makes it an essential part of any weight loss diet program. Fat oxidation is blocked by up to 50% in just 2 weeks, and the tea could also be beneficial for those who suffer from heart ailments, and diabetes. It also prevents toothache, and helps make the skin radiant. You can make Oolong tea for just five minutes—or more. For a stronger cup, just steep it in a cup of hot water for 15 minutes to maximizes the flavor.

4. **Peppermint Tea.** The amazing thing about Peppermint Tea is the

fact that it suppresses the appetite, while it actually speeds up digestion. You have to use the leaves of the peppermint plant to make your tea, since most of the stuff sold in the stores are just green tea infused with peppermint flavor. Remember to add fresh or dried leaves to boiling water, and allow 4 to 5 minutes of steeping. Add some honey, if you want to. Take the tea hot or cold—it's all up to you.

5. **Yerba Mate.** Yerba Mate is responsible for maintaining good cholesterol levels, and has long been known as one of those teas that may prevent cancer. The great about this plant is that it has high antioxidant capacity, which means that it is also rich in polyphenols, which can increase the activity of enzymes that break bad cholesterol down. It's said that it's best to steep the tea in a squash gourd, and a metal straw should be used to drink it, too. You could also use a coffee maker to make the tea in—just put the pod where you usually put coffee grounds.

Precautions:

This herb should be avoided by pregnant and nursing mothers. Those who have a history of alcoholism and substance abuse also need to steer clear of this herb. People with heart problems, diabetes, anxiety and glaucoma should not take this tea since it can aggravate the condition. Keep this away from children since it can cause detrimental effects on their health.

6. **Chamomile.** Chamomile reduces indigestion and nausea and could also calm the mind and soothe the soul—that's why it's often referred as a stress-busting tea. Hyperactive people also benefit from chamomile because it could easily stabilize one's mood, and is perfect for those who suffer from insomnia, as well.

Precautions:

Chamomile acts as a blood thinner so those who are taking medications such as warfarin and other anticoagulants should consult their physician prior to intake. Do not take the tea without assessing the safety of use in conjunction with maintenance medication.

Those who are allergic to plants under the daisy family such as marigold and ragweed should avoid taking chamomile.

Pregnant and nursing women should discuss the potential side effects with their health care provider prior to use of supplements.

7. **Rose Tea.** And of course, there's also Rose Tea, which is best known to prevent and treat dyspepsia! This tea is made from rose buds and flowers and is known to be extremely therapeutic. It contains vitamins A, C, B3, D, and E that could help boost one's metabolism, prevent constipation, and also protect the body against infections. To make the tea, make sure that you first clean the petals with the help of boiling water, then add 2 to 3 cups of the petals into a saucepan and boil for around 5 minutes. Strain and pour before drinking!

Precautions:

Limit intake to less than five cups daily to avoid any potential side effects.

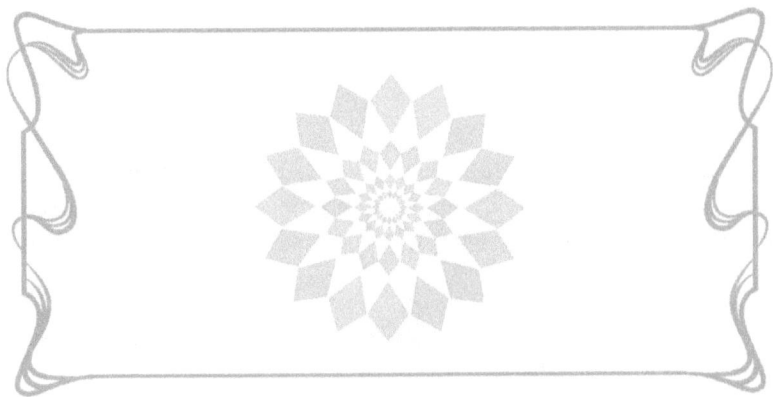

Chapter 13

Diarrhea

Diarrhea is a condition wherein you expel loose and watery stools at a high volume. This is often uncomfortable, uncontrollable and accompanied by stomach cramps and bloating.

There are many reasons for the onset of diarrhea. It's more of a symptom of an infection.

Common causes behind diarrhea are the following:

- Viral or bacterial infection of the gut such as gastroenteritis, food poisoning or stomach flu.
- Food allergies such as lactose intolerance
- Inflammatory Bowel Syndrome (IBS)

In normal cases, diarrhea often resolves on its own after a few days. As the watery stools are expelled, the infection on the gut also clears out.

Natural Remedies

1. Have Some Yogurt

When experiencing diarrhea, both the good and bad bacteria in the gut is flushed out. Yogurt helps by replenishing the number of good bacteria in the gut. Once there's more good bacteria than bad, the diarrhea will subside and gut balance is restored.

Just have a bowl of yogurt each day—add some fruits to get some flavor—or eat with banana and you're all set!

2. Speaking of Bananas, Go Eat Some

Bananas have high pectin content. Pectin is basically water-soluble fiber that reduces diarrhea.

Loose stools contain waste as well as electrolytes (sodium and potassium). These are essential in keeping the water balance in the body, so when you eliminate watery stools you also need to replenish fluids in order to keep the body functional and avoid dehydration. Bananas is a good source of potassium which you need when experiencing bouts of diarrhea.

3. Ginger

The antibacterial properties of ginger help by fighting off the infection in the gut. It can help lessen the symptoms until recovery.

Preparation:
1. Mix ginger juice with honey and lemon juice and drink 3 to 4 times a day—or until your diarrhea is gone.
2. Add a teaspoon of freshly grated ginger with boiling water. Steep for a few minutes, and drink 3 to 4 times a day.

4. Use Diarrhea-Healing Teas

Certain teas could alleviate the effects of diarrhea, as well as ease anxiety which can trigger it. Here are some teas that can give you some relief:

1. **Linden**. Linden is responsible for relaxing nerves and muscles, which of course, prevents stress and calms the mind. Linden Tea is also recommended for people who often suffer from nerve tension, as well as stress-induced headaches. A premade tea can go a long way to reap its benefits.

    Precautions:

    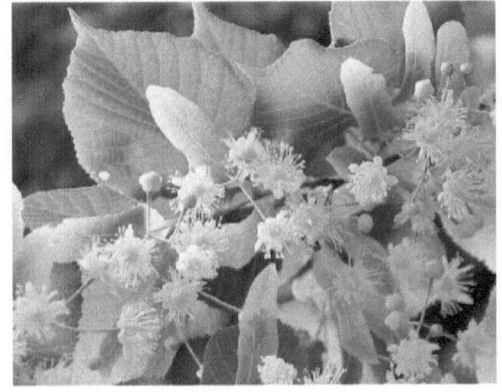

    This is generally safe at recommended dosages. However, those who have heart problems need to consult a physician prior to use since frequent intake of linden can cause heart problems.

2. **Passiflora Incarnate.** This tea reduces headaches that have been brought on by stress and anxiety. Also, it's great for women suffering from PMS and menstrual cramps, and may lessen irritability.

    A good quality premade tea can be a great to have in cases when it might be needed.

    Precautions:

    Avoid using this herb when pregnant and nursing. It's generally safe to use for two months at recommended doses. May interact with maintenance medications such as antiplatelet, anticoagulants, sedatives and monoamine oxidase inhibitors. Do not take in conjunction with any of the medications classified above.

3. **Skullcap.** It's said that no other tea can help muscles relax more than skullcap. It reduces headaches, calms the nerves, and reduces muscle spasms, and prevents muscle tension, as well. Also, women with PMS and menstrual cramps would benefit a lot from this tea, too! It alleviates pain and prevents severe PMS.

    Precautions:

    This herb is not advised for pregnant and nursing women. Avoid taking it at high doses since it can cause neurological symptoms such as twitching, mental confusion, stupor and seizures.

    Chinese skullcap needs to be taken cautiously by those who have diabetes. Those with spleen and stomach problems should avoid taking this herb.

Home Interventions

Here is a simple recipe for an oral rehydrating solution, which can easily be prepared at home:

- 1 glass (240 ml) of water
- 1 tsp. of sugar
- ¼ tsp. of salt

Mix everything until the salt and sugar fully dissolve. Drink in small increments to rehydrate.

When to seek medical assistance:

For severe diarrhea, there is always a danger for dehydration. Always make sure to replenish any fluids lost.

Signs of dehydration include:

Adults:
- Fatigue
- Increased heart rate

- Thirst/dry mouth
- Low urine output
- Headache
- Poor skin turgor

Children:
- Fussiness
- No tears when crying
- Lethargy
- Dry skin
- Poor skin turgor
- Sunken fontanels and eyes (more apparent for severe dehydration)

For adults, diarrhea that is lasts more than three days and accompanied by fever, bloody stools or black and tarry feces indicate a more serious condition and needs further assistance.

For children, you also need to check with your physician if they have a fever for the past 24 hours at a temperature of 102 °F or above. If the stools have blood, mucus or black and tarry, this also requires medical attention. With regards to kids, it's always good to be on the safe side and consult your GP.

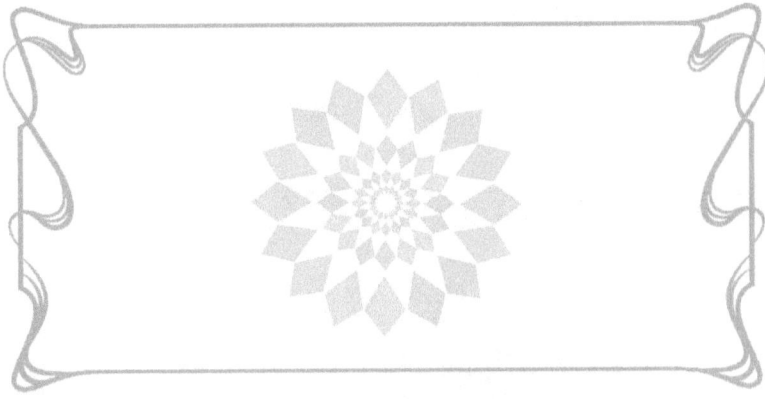

Chapter 14

Vomiting

Vomiting is a forced expulsion of the contents of your stomach through the esophagus and out of the mouth. This is the body's way of removing foreign bodies and gastric irritants.

In most cases, vomiting is a minor ailment that would just go away in its own, especially in cases such as food poisoning or stomach flu. It can also be a sign of something more serious but for the most part I'll only tackle the minor issues that can be addressed at home.

Common causes of vomiting:

Adults:
- Food poisoning
- Pregnancy
- GERD
- Food allergies
- Motion sickness
- Severe pain

Children:

- Gastroenteritis
- Food poisoning

Natural Remedies

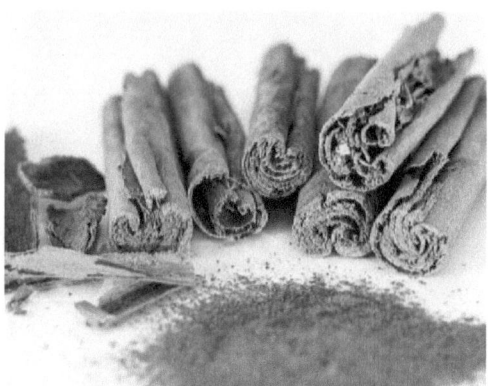

1. Drink Rice Water

Rice water has demulcent properties which help by soothing and coating the stomach lining. This alleviates vomiting and pain from conditions such as gastritis. What you can do is try the following:

1. Boil a cup of rice with 1 ½ cup of water.
2. Strain, and drink just like you would a normal beverage.

2. Cinnamon

Cinnamon has great antibacterial properties which can aid in relieving vomiting from food poisoning. It also known as a carminative, making it effective in combating diarrhea and morning sickness. The catechins in cinnamon help relieve nausea and stimulates the digestive system. Here's what you have to do:

1. Add ½ or 1 teaspoon of cinnamon powder to a cup of boiling water.
2. Steep this mixture for about 15 minutes. You can either strain the mixture or leave it as is if you don't mind the powder.
3. Add a tablespoon of honey, and sip the mixture slowly.

3. Clove

Clove has long been used as a traditional remedy. It is believed to boost enzyme activity and increases metabolic functions. You can chew cloves raw or add some honey to make it more palatable. Since it has antibacterial properties, it may help with the underlying cause of vomiting such as in cases of food poisoning.

4. Peppermint

Mint helps relieve nausea and vomiting my numbing the stomach wall. Studies doesn't support the effect of mint in preventing vomiting during pregnancy but it does help in lessening the discomfort.

Mix mint juice or tea with lemon and honey and drink it to help yourself feel better. Try to drink this at least 2 to 3 times a day, if possible.

5. Fennel

Fennel relaxes the smooth muscles lining the intestinal tract. The bioactive compounds of this herb also helps in expelling gas and reducing bloating.

Mix some crushed fennel seeds with a cup of boiling water, and steep for at least 10 minutes. Strain, and then drink at least once or twice a day. You can also chew a teaspoon of fennel seeds to ease your vomiting.

Precautions:

This should be avoided by pregnant and nursing women. Avoid giving fennel to prepubescent girls since it can cause premature breast development. Fennel affects the metabolic enzymes of some drugs, so it's advisable to check with a provider when taking any maintenance medication.

6. Try Drinking Tea

Once you have calmed down a bit from vomiting, you can try drinking teas that are soothing and rejuvenating so you could regain your strength. These include the following:

1. **Rooibos.** This tea is a well-known remedy in South Africa. It has strong antioxidant properties and has been used for infant colic since the 1970s. It has been tested during that time on local babies with good results. Scientific research hasn't been done to prove the effects of this tea for digestive problems but it is still used widely as a health drink to promote good quality sleep and relieve stress, which is credited to its high flavonoids. The best thing about Rooibos tea is that it inhibits fat cell formation. By drinking Rooibos tea, you'd get to prevent fat cell formation by up to 22%! This way, one's hunger is also suppressed—which leads to fat-burning, as well.

Precautions:

Rooibos affects the hormones in the body, so those with history of breast cancer or hormone related health issues should consult a physician prior to use. This herb mimics estrogen activity so precautions need to be taken for high risk individuals.

Safety for pregnant and nursing women have not yet been established. Avoid this herb if you have liver and kidney issues.

2. **Green Tea.** The thing about Green tea is that it's antioxidant properties help break down fat which boosts energy and hastens the metabolic rate, making sure that the body is regulated. Tannins in tea has astringent properties, which help in reducing toxins in the digestive tract. Green tea generally improves immunity, as well!

Precautions:

Too much tea can cause abdominal pain, nausea and vomiting, so make sure to regulate the amount that you drink.

3. **Chamomile Tea.** This tea has been used traditionally to improve gastric problems, especially digestive issues and hyperacidity. In fact, chamomile oil can be applied on the stomach for relief of colic, flatulence and bloating. The tea takes all these benefits internally.

To make your own chamomile tea, you'll need either fresh or dried chamomile flowers, honey, lemon and apples (optional).

   1. Fill a pot with boiling water.

2. Add freshly washed chamomile flowers or dried ones if that's what you have.
3. Steep for 5 minutes then strain the mixture.
4. Let it cool a bit before adding honey and lemon juice for added flavor.

OPTIONAL: Add some apples while steeping the mixture to infuse a different and delicious flavor. You can release the juice by crushing it while steeping in the pot.

Home Interventions

After a bout of vomiting it's always advised to lie down and rest. For morning sickness, you can eat some dry biscuits or peppermint to help settle your stomach.

Oral Rehydrating solution can be prepared at home by preparing 1 glass filled with water and adding 1 tsp. of sugar and 1/4 tsp. of salt. Mix it well and take small sips to replace lost fluids. You can also buy a premixed pack for this one.

When to seek medical assistance

There are different signs to look for in adults and children, which may give you a clue on whether the condition is minor or requires medical intervention.

Adults:
- Any signs of severe dehydration.
- Persistent vomiting for 24 hours
- Severe stomach pain
- Headache or stiff neck

Children:
- If your child persistently vomiting and unable to hold down fluids in the last 24 hours.
- When they have signs and symptoms of dehydration
- Green colored or bloody vomit

Chapter 15

Nausea

Nausea is the urge to vomit. It can be caused by problems in the gastrointestinal tract or other parts of the body such as the ear.

Nausea usually goes together with vomiting. There are common reasons for feeling nauseous, such as:

Adults:
- motion sickness
- stress (emotional or psychological)
- food poisoning
- exposure to toxins
- indigestion/food intolerance

Children:
- Motion sickness
- Cough
- Overeating
- High fever

Home intervention for nausea is the same for vomiting. Getting lots of rest is important until the sensation or urge to vomit passes. Eat dry food such as biscuits.

Natural Remedies

1. Bananas + Rice + Applesauce + Toast

Sometimes called BRAT, this combination of ingredients can easily calm an upset stomach, and nausea, mainly because they do not contain spices or salt. All of the food items listed above are a great source of carbohydrates. These types of food are easily digested. Just eat them for as long as you're feeling nauseated.
Note: This not advised for long term use, since it is also low in protein, fiber and fat. It isn't a complete meal.

2. Peppermint

Brew some peppermint tea, or eat mint candy, or sniff peppermint extract so you could alleviate the effects of nausea and keep the discomfort at a minimum! If you want, you can even just chew the leaves themselves, too!

3. Jasmine

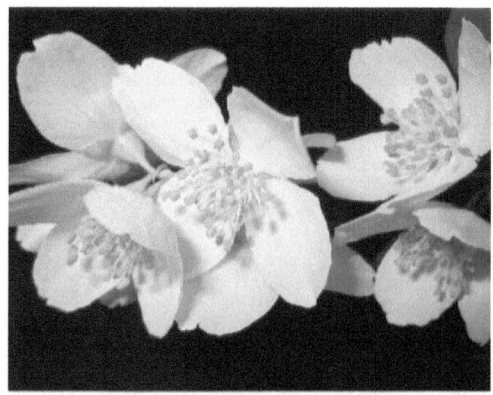

Jasmine Oil is extracted solely from the flowers of the said plant and is also known as "Queen of the Night" because it is best used before sleeping and the flowers are naturally more aromatic at night and is mainly used to bring happiness. Literally, the name "Jasmine" means "Young Girl". It is also known for its healing properties and the fact that it takes care of the reproductive system more than any other oil does.

Jasmine is reputed to prevent the development of stomach ulcer, encourage the production of natural probiotics in the body and aids the digestive process. In high quantities, it can cause gastrointestinal pain and reflux, so this must be taken in moderation. It has antimicrobial properties, making it effective to take when experiencing food poisoning to relieve symptoms. It's an anti-spasmodic, which helps relax the stomach muscles.

You can drink jasmine tea or add jasmine flowers to your beverages for flavor.

Precautions:

This drink is not advisable for pregnant women since it may stimulate the uterine muscles to contract.

You can make Jasmine Oil by doing this:
1. Place jojoba or extra virgin olive oil together with jasmine petals in a jar then put the lid on and shake the mixture thoroughly.
2. Open the jar then pull or bruise the petals then shake again.
3. Place the jar in a sunny place for around 48 hours and make sure to shake the jar every 12 hours. Remove the lid and pour the mixture into another jar. Use muslin cloth as a sieve then pour the mixture back in the jar and leave outside for another 48 hours.
4. Keep the jar in a cool, dry place and use whenever necessary.
5. Use it undiluted then apply 2 to 4 drops on vital points, or inhale directly. You can have it diffused around the room, as well.

4. <u>Ginger</u>

Ginger is one of the most popular remedies for nausea. Several studies have been conducted to test the efficacy of this spice as an antiemetic. It has been tested on nausea caused by chemotherapy, post-operative state and pregnancy. The results concluded that ginger is an effective remedy when compared to placebo pills. There were some instances where this spice worked equally well with metoclopramide.

Preparation:
1. Put 2 tbsp. of ginger powder in a tub filled with warm water. Get in the tub and soak in the water for a good 10 minutes, and then go to sleep after patting your body dry. Use a blanket to cover yourself with completely.
2. Add a teaspoon of freshly grated ginger with boiling water. Steep

for a few minutes, and drink 3 to 4 times a day.

5.   Lavender

The most well-known essential oil, Lavender has antibacterial and anti-viral properties which are essential for treating bites, scrapes and stings. It can be used on its own without carrier oil which makes it one of the most accessible oils on the planet. In Latin, Lavender literally means "to wash"—which means that using it that help you clear off unnecessary toxins in your system and make you feel better about yourself. It is also said that Lavender promotes clarity of mind and improves one's intuition, too.

Lavender helps by settling the stomach and can stop nausea. It has antibacterial properties, which can help ease food poisoning and relieve some of its symptoms.

You can use lavender essential oil by rubbing some of it on your solar plexus when needed. You can also diffuse the oil to get the same effect.

Precautions:

This isn't advisable for pregnant women, especially in the first trimester.

To make Lavender Oil, you can follow the steps below:

1.   Make sure that you use fresh lavender petals and stems. You may plant some lavender so you could harvest what you need in the future.
2.   Clip the flowers into small pieces then bend the stems so they could easily fit in the jar. Fill up the jar with both the stems and petals but make sure not to stuff it and leave some room to breathe.
3.   Pour some extra virgin olive oil into the jar then put a stopper so there would be no air pockets between the plant and the oil.
4.   Seal the jar and let it sit for around a month. Place it somewhere with direct sunlight then make sure to shake it a bit daily so the oil would be well-mixed.
5.   After a month, remove the stopper then pour the contents into another jar. Make sure that you are able to transfer all of the oil. Throw excess lavender away and store the jar in a cool, dry place.

Use it by applying at least 2 to 4 drops on vital points, or have it diffused around the room.

Home Intervention

Use a Heating Pad
When you feel nauseous from pain and menstrual cramps, then a heating pad can do wonders. If you don't have a heating pad, you can simply use a hot water bottle as an alternative.

When to seek medical assistance

Here are few warning signs to look:

Children:
- Projectile vomiting
- Fever of more than 100 °F - 102 °F
- Showing sign of dehydration with no urine output for the last six hours
- Has been vomiting for two hours (below six years old) and 24 hours (six and above).
- Lethargic

Adults:
- Lethargy and confusion
- Severe pain in the abdominal area
- Increased respiration rate, blood pressure and pulse
- Fever of more than 102 °F
- Severe headaches with stiff neck

MARY CONRAD

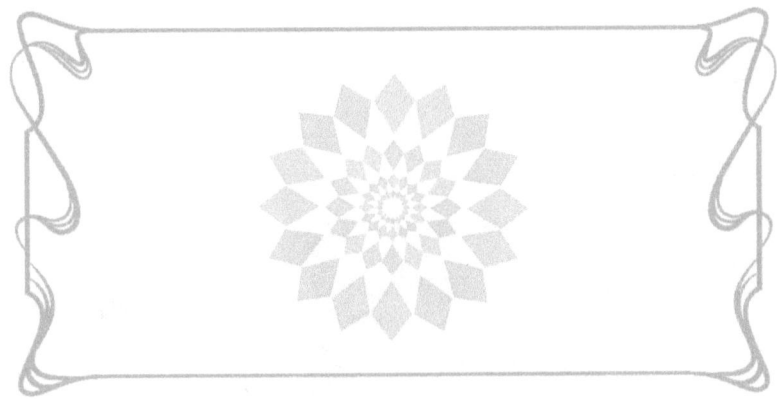

Chapter 16

Cuts

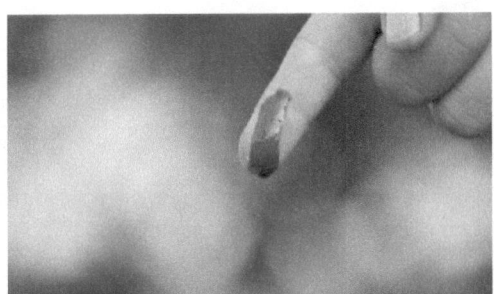
Cuts are minor wounds that refer to a small breach in the skin's integrity. It can be as small as a scrape on the knee to a shallow cut from a kitchen knife. A cut is considered minor if it doesn't require stitches or any medical attention. If the cut is less than 2 cm. and isn't deep, then there shouldn't be any problems. Bleeding usually stops after a few minutes when pressure is applied.

The danger of minor cuts is usually in the form of infection. Since these cuts often seem harmless, it's easy to forget that they're there.

Signs of infection include:

- Swelling, redness and pain in the wound
- Pus is in the wound or any smelly discharge
- High fever
- Swollen lymph glands

Natural Remedies

1. <u>Calendula</u>

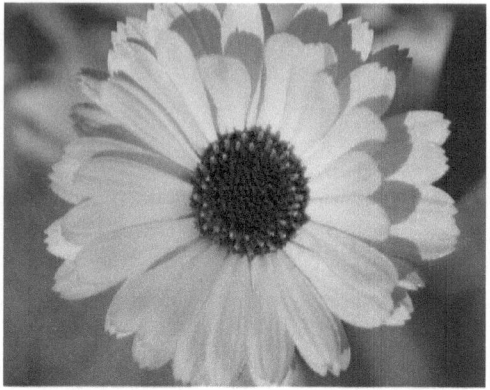

This plant helps heal cuts by increasing the blood flow and oxygen in the affected area. This in turn helps the body regenerate new tissues and cells. It can be used to keep the skin hydrated as well as keeping it firm and supple. It can be used for minor infection and is commonly used topically.

You can make your own calendula essential oil by using calendula flowers and olive oil.

1. In glass jar, add the calendula flowers. Make sure that the flowers are dry and without excess moisture. Pour olive oil on the flowers until the oil is about an inch above the flowers, soaking it through.
2. Place in a sunny area, and stir every 12 hours.
3. After six weeks, strain the mixture and transfer the oil in a dark glass bottle. Store it in a cool dry place.

Calendula Salve

You can use this for minor cuts, but make sure that the wound has already closed. It wouldn't be a good idea to apply it on an open wound for safety reasons.

- 4 ounces of Calendula essential oil
- 1/2 ounce of beeswax

Melt the beeswax and add the essential oil. Once mixed and completely melted, transfer in a glass container. Make sure that the mixture has cooled before closing the cap.

Calendula Wash

- Sea Salt
- Calendula essential oil
- Water

1. Take some warm water (240 ml) and add 10 drops of essential oil. Add sea salt and mix thoroughly. You may also add a few drops of lavender oil for added fragrance and health benefits.
2. Transfer to a mist bottle use.

You can use this to disinfect small wounds.

2. Honey

Raw honey has great medical property at dates back to Ancient Greece and Egypt. It has strong antibacterial properties that inhibit the growth of bacteria. In wound healing, it works by drawing out the moisture from the environment, which dehydrates the bacteria. It also increases the healing process by creating a conducive environment for tissue growth. and repair.

To use honey, coat the affected area once daily.

3. Roman Chamomile

It is said that Roman Chamomile Oil promotes inner peace and may help remind someone of days gone by because of its nostalgic and sweet scent. Roman Chamomile is also one of the most popular and beneficial essential oils around as it is truly calming and relaxing and promotes holistic healing.

Literally, Chamomile means "Greek Apple" which is said to resonate one's childhood and innocence, also making it one of the best essential oils for babies. The topmost flowers are used to create the essential oil.

Traditionally, chamomile has been used as a wound healing agent for quite a long time. It works by speeding up the epithelialization of the wound and keeping it dry. It has antibacterial properties, which can help prevent wound infection.

You can create an infusion from chamomile flowers and use that to dab gently on cuts.

1. In a teapot add one ounce of fresh chamomile flowers (ratio is one ounce per one cup of water).
2. Pour boiling water, making sure to soak the flowers through. Cover the pot right away. Let it infuse for 15 minutes so the oils will disperse into the water and pot.
3. After, you can use the liquid to dab on the affected area.

Precautions:

Make sure the liquid isn't hot during application.

You can make Chamomile Oil by following the instructions below:

1. Buy some dried chamomile flowers. If you have access to fresh ones in your garden, that would also work. Discard any debris or sand/soil and wash it in cool running water.
2. Place the flowers on a cutting board to dry them completely.
3. Next, sterilize a glass jar then pour some olive oil into it up to at least ½ inch near the top.
4. Add the chamomile flowers then stir until each flower is covered submerged in oil. Put the lid on tightly.
5. Place the jar in an area under direct sunlight then leave it be for around 2 weeks or until flowers are spent.
6. Transfer the oil into another clean jar then sieve out any flowers left behind. Strain until no more flowers are left.
7. Stir well and store in a cool, dry place.

To use, simply apply at least 2 to 4 drops to your ankles, wrists, and other vital points. You could also choose to have it diffused around the room. Direct inhalation may be good, too.

4. Apply the Following

Make mixtures out of the following and apply them on your cuts:

1. **Tea Tree Oil.** Using tea tree oil as a wash for minor wounds is easy and effective. This oil has antiseptic, antibacterial, antiviral, anti-inflammatory and antifungal properties. It also aids in tissue regeneration. With all these benefits, you can use the oil to clean a

cut. It's best to use a diluted form of the oil as a wound wash since it'll sting less and safer compared to using the essential oil directly.

Tea Tree Oil Wound Wash

Take a cup of previously boiled water (make sure that it has cooled). Add two drops of tea tree oil. Mix it. You can add a pinch of sea salt or Epsom salt to help diffuse the oil in water. Dip a cloth in the mixture and use it wash the cuts and scrapes. Get some tea tree oil and use absorbent cotton to help you apply it on the affected area.

2. **Spinach**. Spinach is also high in vitamins, minerals and fiber. It's high phytonutrient content is responsible for the anti-inflammatory and anti-cancer properties of this vegetable. Get spinach leaves and wash them. Break into veins or ridges and place where you have been bruised.

3. **Oatmeal.** Cook some oatmeal and then directly apply it to where you have been bruised so that inflammation will be relieved.

4. **Marshmallow Root.** Mix it with equal parts of flaxseed in a pot of boiling water. Use clean cloth to dip into the mixture, and then apply it to the bruised area. This also works for sprains, earaches, and toothaches, as well.

5. **Lettuce.** Similar to cucumbers, lettuce is a rich source of vitamin A, which helps trigger the synthesis of collagen in the body; thereby promoting wound healing. It also has anti-inflammatory properties that may also prove useful. Place some cool lettuce on abrasions that are raw, cover with cloth, and have it enclosed for an hour or two.

6. **Fenugreek.** Get some crushed fenugreek seeds and add to your bath. Not only does it ease bruising, it also prevents congestion from happening in most parts of your body. Use it with olive oil for better effects, as well.

7. **Cucumber.** Cucumber is not only cool and delicious but it can help in wound healing by increasing the rate of collagen production in the skin. It's a rich source of vitamin A and silica, which assists the body in forming connective tissues.

Eat raw cucumbers to get the maximum benefits of this vegetable.

5. Cayenne Pepper

Cayenne pepper can help stop the wound from bleeding, but use it as a last resort. If the bleeding is minor enough, use direct pressure on the wound to staunch the bleeding. In cases where there's a bit more blood and applying pressure isn't helping then you can try sprinkling cayenne pepper on the open wound. Take note that this is only for minor wounds, and it could sting but it has also proven to effective. It also helps disinfect the wound because it has antibacterial and antifungal properties. For cayenne wound wash you can try the doing the steps below:

1. In a glass of water, mix 1 tsp. of cayenne pepper. Dip a wash cloth in the mixture.
2. Apply directly on affected area for 10 to 12 seconds

6. Shred Some Potatoes

Yes, potatoes can heal wounds!

Potatoes have shown to be effective in wound healing from burns, but it is also used for minor cuts to enhance the rate of cell recovery and prevent the development of abscess. Shred a couple of potatoes and just apply the shredded potatoes to your cuts at least 4 times a day so that the inflammation would be reduced, and so you can be sure that your cuts would not be infected.

Home Interventions

The first thing you have to do is make sure that the wound is clean of any dirt or debris. Place the wound under cool running water to help wash out it out. Once clean, apply pressure to stop the bleeding. You can use a clean towel or handkerchief. Place it on the wounded area and lightly apply pressure. In a few minutes, the bleeding will likely stop. Using water or an antiseptic, you can clean the surrounding area to prevent infection. Tap the area dry. You can choose to apply a dressing for open wounds to keep out any moisture foreign bodies. Just make sure to clean this once daily and reapply the dressing until the wound completely closes over.

For deeper wounds, you can help reduce the bleeding by elevating the affected area before giving first aid. After which, you can assess whether or not it requires stitches or not.

When to seek medical attention

In cases where the cut is caused by an animal bite, it's always best to have it checked. If the wound is bleeding heavily and isn't staunched by pressure, there's a possibility that a blood vessel may have been cut and this may need stitches and medical assistance. If any foreign body is lodged in the wound, it would need to be removed and disinfected properly.

MARY CONRAD

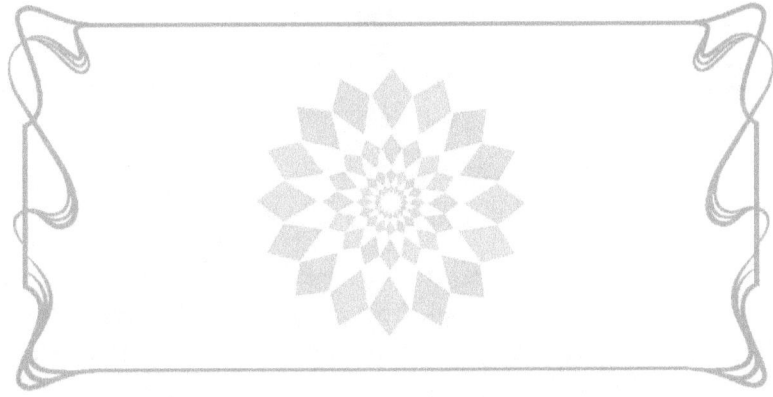

Chapter 17

Nail Fungus

Nail fungus is a condition wherein the opportunistic pathogens (specifically fungus) than live on our skin starts taking over an area causing it to grow and thrive. It often appears as a yellow or white spot under the fingernails or toes.

The reason this happens are varied but still quite common, such as: lack of circulation in the area, persistent exposure to moisture and small open wounds that become pathways for infection. Nail fungus is actually more common in the toenails since it provides a more conducive environment for fungal growth (a moist, dark environment when wearing closed shoes).

Those who have low immunity or problems with circulation are often more at risk for developing nail fungus. For those who have diabetes, it's best to consult a physician when you think you have nail fungus to avoid any complications that it could cause.

Natural Remedies

1. **Make Use of Baking Soda**

This remedy works by creating an alkaline environment where fungus have trouble growing in. Continued usage will kill off the fungus and heal the nail. It may take a few weeks for the nail to fully heal. Once the yellowing subsides and the nail thins down to normal, you can stop this regimen.

Preparation:

1. Mix ¼ cup of peroxide, ½ cup of baking soda, 4 cups of water, and ½ cup of Epsom salt, and mix all these with ¼ cup of white vinegar.

2. Soak your nail in this solution for a few minutes, and then use a cotton ball and dip it into this solution.

3. Tape the cotton ball to the nail for just 1 to 10 hours each day, for 4 weeks.

You can also just wash your hands every day in a combination of warm water and baking soda. Do it twice a day.

2. **Olive Leaf Extract**

The phenolic compounds of olive leaf extract inhibit the growth of fungi. This is usually taken as a supplement but due to its detoxifying qualities it may cause some discomfort when taken at first. For chronic fungal infections, this might be a helpful alternative.

Apply the extract on the affected area twice daily. Massage it for maximum benefits since improving the circulation in the area will also hasten healing.

Precautions:

Pregnant and breastfeeding mothers should not take this as a supplement without proper medical guidance.

3. <u>ACV</u>

ACV works by increasing the number of good bacteria in the skin. The mixture of acid and enzymes help in fighting off the infection.

One more thing you can do with ACV is mix it with Epsom salt and 6 parts of hot water. Try to let it cool first before using it. Soak your feet in the mixture for at least 2 to 3 times each day so the fungi would be killed.

4. <u>Lavender Oil</u>

The Lavender oil you've made earlier will be useful against nail fungus. Just put a few drops of it on your affected nails and cover your nails with socks made from wool, and not made of other fibers that may irritate both the skin and the nails. Continue doing so each day until you are healed.

5. <u>Coconut Oil</u>

You can also try using coconut oil because it's able to penetrate cell walls—and even fight yeast infections, such as Candida. It breaks through the cells walls of the fungus allowing the intercellular fluids to leak which kills the cell. Apply some oil to the affected areas as needed.

6. <u>Oregano</u>

This herb has been used as an old folk remedy in the Mediterranean for eons. It has great antibacterial, antiviral and antifungal properties, mainly due to two compounds —thymol and carvacrol. It also aids in keeping the digestive system healthy. It's very effective but also very potent.

To use for nail fungus, mix one drop of oregano essential oil with one ounce of olive or almond oil. Apply a drop of the mixture on the affected area.

Precautions:

Pregnant women should avoid taking the oil since it promotes menstruation. Those who have iron deficiency, should contact their physician prior to use.

7. <u>Tea Tree Oil</u>

This is a tried and tested remedy for nail fungus. Tea tree has great antifungal properties. It also alters the environment of the affected area by drying it out.

Since tea tree oil is relatively mild, you can directly use one drop of the essential oil on the affected nail. Make sure that the oil is absorbed in the nail bed. Trim any excess nail so the oil can be absorbed properly. Do this three times daily until the nail fungus disappears. This will be apparent when the nail color returns to normal and no yellow or white tinge is seen.

If you haven't tried tea tree oil yet, make sure to dilute the first dose with carrier oil such as coconut oil and almond oil.

8. <u>Cinnamon oil</u>

Cinnamon oil is a potent antifungal agent but it can also be irritating to the skin. To use this oil, mix one drop of 100% cinnamon bark oil with ¼ cup of carrier oil. Test this on your skin to ensure that it is tolerated before using the mixture further. Use one drop of the mixture on the affected area once daily.

Home Intervention

When applying any of the remedies above, it's best to cut the thick nails so the oil or powder can reach deeper into the nail. You can soak the affected area with water to soften the nail and prepare it for cutting. Be careful not to injure yourself while doing this.

- Disinfect your footwear to avoid recurrent infection.

- Keep feet dry or wear absorbent socks

- Wearing closed shoes at long intervals may lead to recurrence of infection

- Get rid of old shoes.

When to seek medical help for nail fungus

1. When you see signs of infection such as:

    - Swelling, redness, inflammation and pain

- Experiencing fever over 104°F

- Yellowish discharge from the affected area

2. When the fungus is spreading to the skin or other nails.

3. When there's pain and discomfort in the area

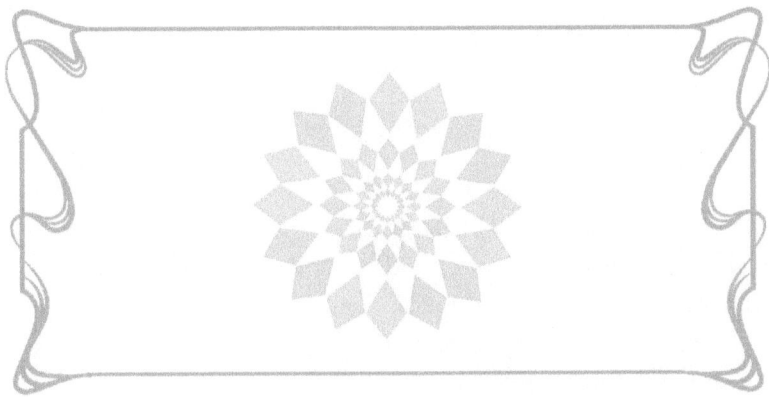

Chapter 18

Minor Burns

A burn occurs when there is damage to skin which causes the cells to die. Minor burns are burns which do not need medical attention, such as a first degree burn and mild second degree burns.

First degree burns affect the top layer of the skin. It's marked by redness, pain and swelling.

Second degree burns affect the first to layers of the skin. This usually leads to blister formation, redness, swelling and pain in the burn area.

Third degree burns are severe burns that extend as far as the muscles. It usually shows some charring, leaves a white waxy color to the burn area, leathery texture and dark brown color.

Natural Remedies

1. **Aloe Vera**

Aloe Vera has been scientifically proven to assist in wound healing, especially with burns. Its effect extends to both first degree and second degree burns and has shown significant anti-inflammatory and wound healing properties. This is on top of its antibacterial properties, which also reduces the risk of infection to the wounded area.

To use aloe vera for burns, just cut off a portion of the leaf. The size would depend on the size of the burn. Scrape of the gel from the leaf and apply on the affected area.

2. **Coconut Oil**

A certain study used coconut oil in the treatment for burns and found that the oil assists in wound healing. The fatty acids, antioxidant and antibacterial properties are the reasons behind its effectiveness.

For application, you can use either cool coconut oil (solid form) and apply it on the affected area. If you have the liquid form of the oil, you can also apply it lightly on the wound to promote healing.

3. **Honey**

Honey is one of the best remedies for healing wounds. It's antibacterial and anti-inflammatory properties help in cell regeneration and even reduces scar tissue formation. It increases the formation of new blood vessels and skin cells which make skin grafting unnecessary.

To use honey, spread a generous amount of honey in a clean gauze. Spread it well, making sure the honey would be able to cover the burn area. Once done, apply the gauze to the injury. Change the dressing every four hours.

4. <u>Plantain</u>

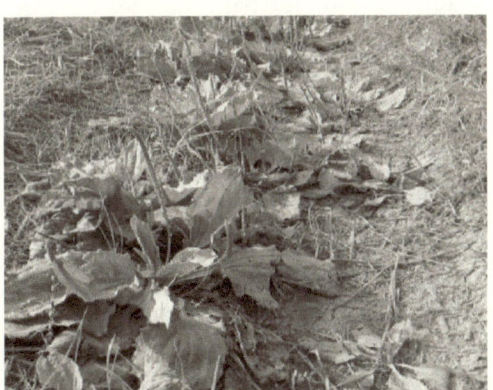 Plantain leaf has been used for centuries as a natural remedy for a number of ailments. One study sought to discover the actual healing properties of the leaf. The results indicated that the leaf contains anti-inflammatory, analgesic, wound healing, antioxidants, mild antibacterial and immune system modulating properties. All of these contribute to its healing effect as well as back up its uses in herbal medicine.

Take some plantain leaves and crush it until a paste is formed. Apply directly on the affected area and keep it there until it dries. Once dry, the plantain paste needs to be replaced. Continue the treatment until relief is felt.

5.   Raw Potato

According to old Chinese remedies, raw potatoes help in minor burn by drawing out the heat in the affected area. Although no studies back up this particular remedy, many have tried it with great results.

Right after the burn injury, wash the area. Take a fresh potato (juicy is best!) and peel it. Mash it to release the juices and apply it on the affected area. Leave it on for about 15-20 minutes or until the pain subsides.

6.   Lavender Essential Oil

Lavender oil has proven effective in healing wounds and reducing pain. Although there are few studies that prove the effectiveness of this oil for wound treatment, there has been a long history of its use for wound healing. One study proved that lavender oil mixed with water managed to alleviate discomfort caused by episiotomy.

To use this oil for wound care, prepare 500 ml of water and add five drops of the essential oil. Apply to the affected area.

Another method is by adding one drop of lavender essential oil in one tablespoon of honey. Spread it on the injury and reapply every three hours.

Home Interventions

Place the injured area under cool running water for few minutes. For chemical burns, let it stay under the spray for about 10-15 minutes. Avoid placing ice in the area, since it can cause further injury. You can place aloe vera cream in the area to help soothe the burn and keep infections at bay.

When to seek medical assistance

It's important to note that medical assistance depend on the location and extensiveness of the injury. For minor burns caused by electrocutions and chemicals or larger than two inches, it's advised to have it checked especially if it's located in the hands, joints, foot, face, groin, buttocks and hip.

If the burn injury encompasses a large area of the skin, always seek medical aid to avoid complication such as infection and dehydration.

MARY CONRAD

Conclusion

Hopefully, you've learned about various home remedies that you can use for minor medical emergencies. This way, you can easily help yourself or any of your family members in case these problems happen. After all, it's always a good idea to be prepared!

No matter how careful we are these minor conditions will happen over time. The best we can do is prepare and have a great reference handy to keep ourselves aware. We don't always need to rush to the hospital. Let the first line of care begin at home. I've found that these remedies, no matter how common can help ease our discomfort from minor ailments. Always remember to monitor either yourself or your loved ones when ill to avoid panic when complications arise.

Finally, if you have enjoyed this book, please take time to post a review on Amazon. It will be greatly appreciated.

Follow me on Twitter: @AuthorMConrad

Also, please like my Facebook page to get the latest news on my next book.

If you have any suggestions or specific natural remedies that you want to have researched and written, shoot me an email at authormaryconrad@gmail.com. I'm always on the lookout for great new topics to write about. :)

Have a great day!

Thank you for taking a step towards health with me today! ☺

Author Biography

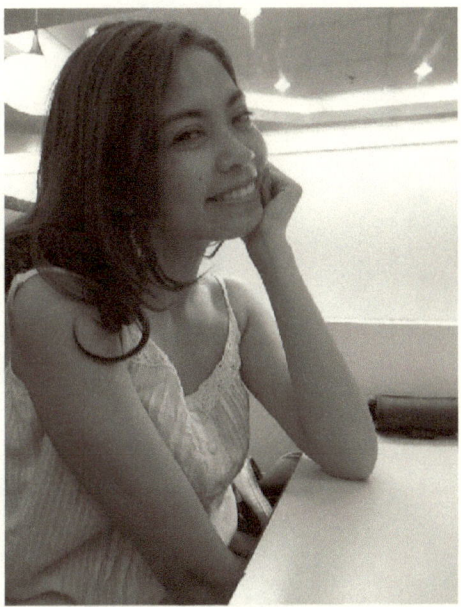

Mary Conrad is a Registered Nurse, who has a strong interest in natural remedies. As a mother, she believes in a holistic approach to health and well-being. Even though she graduated in the health profession, which usually advocates pharmaceutical medication, she believes that prevention is the best step towards health. Backed with scientific research, she wrote these books for both personal information and for others who share the same passion for holistic wellness. It's all about knowing the best natural ways to prevent disease and remedy current health problems. Like every health care provider, she believes in doing no harm, and promoting health. Take a step towards health, and towards nature.

MARY CONRAD

References:

Ruiz, M. E. (2010). Risks of self-medication practices. Current drug safety, 5(4), 315-323.http://www.ncbi.nlm.nih.gov/pubmed/20615179

World Health Organization. (1998). The Role of the pharmacist in self-care and self-medication: report of the 4th WHO Consultative Group on the Role of the Pharmacist, The Hague, The Netherlands, 26-28 August 1998. http://apps.who.int/medicinedocs/en/d/Jwhozip32e/3.3.html

Herbal medicine. (n.d.). Retrieved July 21, 2016, from https://umm.edu/health/medical/altmed/treatment/herbal-medicine

Paul, I. M., Beiler, J., McMonagle, A., Shaffer, M. L., Duda, L., & Berlin, C. M. (2007). Effect of honey, dextromethorphan, and no treatment on nocturnal cough and sleep quality for coughing children and their parents. Archives of pediatrics & adolescent medicine, 161(12), 1140-1146. http://www.ncbi.nlm.nih.gov/pubmed/18056558

Lemon Juice, Honey & Hot Water for a Cough. (2015). Retrieved July 23, 2016, from http://www.livestrong.com/article/271163-lemon-juice-honey-hot-water-for-a-cough/

Med-Health.net. (n.d.). Retrieved July 23, 2016, from http://www.med-health.net/Honey-And-Lemon-For-Cough.html

Sharma, K. D., Karki, S., Thakur, N. S., & Attri, S. (2012). Chemical composition, functional properties and processing of carrot—a review. Journal of food science and technology, 49(1), 22-32. http://www.ncbi.nlm.nih.gov/pmc/articles/PMC3550877/#!po=4.41176
Carrots: Health Benefits, Nutritional Information. (n.d.). Retrieved July 23, 2016, from http://www.medicalnewstoday.com/articles/270191.php

Using Turmeric for Cough. (n.d.). Retrieved July 23, 2016, from http://www.turmericforhealth.com/turmeric-benefits/using-turmeric-for-cough

TURMERIC: Uses, Side Effects, Interactions and Warnings - WebMD. (n.d.). Retrieved July 23, 2016, from http://www.webmd.com/vitamins-supplements/ingredientmono-662-turmeric.aspx?activeingredientid=662

Grape seed extract as a treatment for asthma. (n.d.). Retrieved July 23,

2016, from http://www.emaxhealth.com/11631/grape-seed-extract-treatment-asthma

Ginger: Uses and Risks. (n.d.). Retrieved July 23, 2016, from http://www.webmd.com/vitamins-and-supplements/ginger-uses-and-risks?page=2

Khalid, N., Suleria, H. A. R., & Ahmed, I. Pineapple Juice.

Common cold (n.d.). Retrieved July 23, 2016, from http://www.nhs.uk/conditions/Cold-common/Pages/Introduction.aspx

Flu or Cold? Know the Differences. (n.d.). Retrieved July 23, 2016, from http://www.webmd.com/cold-and-flu/cold-guide/flu-cold-symptoms?page=2

What Caused This Bug Bite? (n.d.). Retrieved July 23, 2016, from http://www.healthline.com/health/bug-bites

Insect bites and stings - Treatment. (n.d.). Retrieved July 23, 2016, from http://www.nhs.uk/Conditions/Bites-insect/Pages/Treatment.aspx

Weinick, R. M., Burns, R. M., & Mehrotra, A. (2010). Many emergency department visits could be managed at urgent care centers and retail clinics. Health Affairs, 29(9), 1630-1636.

22 Natural Sore Throat Remedies to Help Soothe the Pain. (2013). Retrieved July 23, 2016, from http://everydayroots.com/sore-throat-remedies

20 Home Remedies for Cuts. (2007). Retrieved July 23, 2016, from http://health.howstuffworks.com/wellness/natural-medicine/home-remedies/home-remedies-for-cuts.htmhttp://homeremediesforlife.com/nail-fungus/

20 Home Remedies for Bruises - Home Remedies - Natural & Herbal Cures Made at Home. (n.d.). Retrieved July 23, 2016, from http://homeremedyshop.com/20-home-remedies-for-bruises/

15 Natural Home Remedies for Wounds | Live Love Fruit. (2014). Retrieved July 23, 2016, from http://livelovefruit.com/15-natural-home-remedies-for-wounds/

40 Home Remedies for Bruises. (n.d.). Retrieved July 23, 2016, from

http://midnightremedies.com/53-1-bruises.htmlhttp://theheartysoul.com/insect-bites-essential-oils/

7 Natural Remedies for Allergy Relief | Wellness Mama. (n.d.). Retrieved July 23, 2016, from http://wellnessmama.com/8370/allergy-relief-remedies/

4 Natural Remedies for Nausea. (n.d.). Retrieved July 23, 2016, from http://www.everydayhealth.com/digestive-health/four-natural-remedies-for-nausea.aspx

The Latest On AXS. (n.d.). Retrieved July 23, 2016, from http://www.examiner.com/article/ten-easy-cures-for-diarrhea

10 Amazing Home Remedies for Vomiting. (n.d.). Retrieved July 23, 2016, from http://www.findhomeremedy.com/10-amazing-home-remedies-for-vomiting/

9 Herbal Remedies For Indigestion. (n.d.). Retrieved July 23, 2016, from http://www.findhomeremedy.com/herbal-remedies-for-indigestion/

7 Natural Remedies for Sore Throats. (n.d.). Retrieved July 23, 2016, from http://www.healthline.com/health/cold-flu/sore-throat-natural-remedies#LicoriceRoot3

6 Natural Upset Stomach Remedies. (n.d.). Retrieved July 23, 2016, from http://www.healthline.com/health/digestive-health/natural-upset-stomach-remedies#3

Herbal Teas for Diarrhea. (2015). Retrieved July 23, 2016, from http://www.livestrong.com/article/110772-herbal-teas-good-diarrhea/

Sprains and strains. (n.d.). Retrieved July 23, 2016, from http://www.mayoclinic.org/diseases-conditions/sprains-and-strains/basics/lifestyle-home-remedies/con-20020958

Top 10 Home Remedies To Get Rid Of Toenail Fungus Fast. (2014). Retrieved July 23, 2016, from http://www.naturallivingideas.com/top-10-natural-remedies-for-toenail-fungus/

The 9 Very Best Essential Oils For Treating Colds And Flu. (n.d.). Retrieved July 23, 2016, from http://www.offthegridnews.com/alternative-health/the-9-very-best-essential-oils-for-treating-colds-and-flu/

12 Natural Allergy Remedies that Provide Relief | Reader's Digest. (n.d.). Retrieved July 23, 2016, from http://www.rd.com/health/conditions/12-natural-allergy-remedies-that-provide-relief/

My Favorite Teas for Bloating, IBS, and Regularity. (n.d.). Retrieved July 23, 2016, from http://www.spinachandyoga.com/my-favorite-teas-for-bloating-ibs-and-regularity/

Home Remedies for Fever | Top 10 Home Remedies. (2014). Retrieved July 23, 2016, from http://www.top10homeremedies.com/home-remedies/home-remedies-fever.html

Home Remedies for Common Cold | Top 10 Home Remedies. (2012). Retrieved July 23, 2016, from http://www.top10homeremedies.com/home-remedies/home-remedies-for-common-cold.html

Home Remedies for Vomiting | Top 10 Home Remedies. (2012). Retrieved July 23, 2016, from http://www.top10homeremedies.com/home-remedies/home-remedies-for-vomiting.html

Home Remedies for a Sprained Ankle | Top 10 Home Remedies. (2014). Retrieved July 23, 2016, from http://www.top10homeremedies.com/home-remedies/home-remedies-sprained-ankle.html

12 Flu and Cold Natural Remedies. (n.d.). Retrieved July 23, 2016, from http://www.webmd.com/cold-and-flu/12-tips-prevent-colds-flu-1

Ankri, S., & Mirelman, D. (1999). Antimicrobial properties of allicin from garlic. Microbes and infection, 1(2), 125-129.

12 Home Remedies for the Cold: Nasal Spray, Steam, & More. (n.d.). Retrieved July 23, 2016, from http://www.webmd.com/cold-and-flu/cold-guide/cold-remedies

Home Remedies for Insect Bites and Stings and Spider Bites. (n.d.). Retrieved July 23, 2016, from http://www.webmd.com/first-aid/tc/insect-bites-and-stings-and-spider-bites-home-treatment

9 Genius Ways To Relieve Bug Bites. (2014). Retrieved July 23, 2016, from http://www.womenshealthmag.com/health/bug-bite-relief

Home Remedies for Dyspepsia | Organic Facts. (2009). Retrieved July 23, 2016, from https://www.organicfacts.net/home-remedies/home-remedies-for-dyspepsia.html

Bruises: Causes, Treatments, Prevention. (n.d.). Retrieved July 23, 2016, from http://www.webmd.com/skin-problems-and-treatments/guide/bruises-article?page=2

What are bruises? (n.d.). Retrieved July 23, 2016, from http://www.nhs.uk/chq/Pages/1057.aspx?CategoryID=72

Sprain: First aid. (n.d.). Retrieved July 23, 2016, from http://www.mayoclinic.org/first-aid/first-aid-sprain/basics/art-20056622

Sprains and strains. (n.d.). Retrieved July 23, 2016, from http://www.nhs.uk/conditions/Sprains/Pages/Introduction.aspx

Sprains and Strains: MedlinePlus. (n.d.). Retrieved July 23, 2016, from https://www.nlm.nih.gov/medlineplus/sprainsandstrains.html

Fever. (n.d.). Retrieved July 23, 2016, from http://www.mayoclinic.org/diseases-conditions/fever/basics/causes/con-20019229

Fever Facts: High Temperature Causes and Treatments. (n.d.). Retrieved July 23, 2016, from http://www.webmd.com/first-aid/fevers-causes-symptoms-treatments?page=1

First Aid You Should Know: How to Treat Allergic Reaction. (n.d.). Retrieved July 23, 2016, from http://www.healthline.com/health/allergies/allergic-reaction-treatment#Symptoms2

Allergies. (n.d.). Retrieved July 23, 2016, from http://www.nhs.uk/conditions/Allergies/Pages/Introduction.aspx

Dyspepsia Causes, Symptoms, Treatments, & More. (n.d.). Retrieved July 23, 2016, from http://www.webmd.com/digestive-disorders/tc/dyspepsia-topic-overview

Indigestion (Dyspepsia, Upset Stomach) Symptoms, Treatment, Causes - What causes dyspepsia (indigestion)? - MedicineNet. (n.d.). Retrieved July 23, 2016, from http://www.medicinenet.com/dyspepsia/page4.htm

What causes diarrhea? 87 possible conditions. (n.d.). Retrieved July 23, 2016, from http://www.healthline.com/symptom/diarrhea

Diarrhea. (n.d.). Retrieved July 23, 2016, from http://www.mayoclinic.org/diseases-conditions/diarrhea/basics/definition/con-20014025

Nausea and vomiting - adults: MedlinePlus Medical Encyclopedia. (n.d.). Retrieved July 23, 2016, from https://www.nlm.nih.gov/medlineplus/ency/article/003117.htm

Vomiting in children and babies. (n.d.). Retrieved July 23, 2016, from http://www.nhs.uk/conditions/vomiting-children-babies/Pages/Introduction.aspx

Nausea and Vomiting. (n.d.). Retrieved July 23, 2016, from http://www.healthline.com/health/nausea-and-vomiting#EmergencyCare3

Cuts and grazes (n.d.). Retrieved July 23, 2016, from http://www.nhs.uk/conditions/Cuts-and-grazes/Pages/Introduction.aspx

Nail fungus. (n.d.). Retrieved July 23, 2016, from http://www.mayoclinic.org/diseases-conditions/nail-fungus/basics/complications/con-20019319

Burns: Types, Treatments, and More. (n.d.). Retrieved July 23, 2016, from http://www.healthline.com/health/burns#Second-degreeburn5

Minor burns - aftercare: MedlinePlus Medical Encyclopedia. (n.d.). Retrieved July 23, 2016, from https://www.nlm.nih.gov/medlineplus/ency/patientinstructions/000662.htm

Maenthaisong, R., Chaiyakunapruk, N., Niruntraporn, S., & Kongkaew, C. (2007). The efficacy of aloe vera used for burn wound healing: a systematic review. burns, 33(6), 713-718.

Somboonwong, J., Thanamittramanee, S., Jariyapongskul, A., &

Patumraj, S. (2000). Therapeutic effects of Aloe vera on cutaneous microcirculation and wound healing in second degree burn model in rats. Journal of the Medical Association of Thailand= Chotmaihet thangphaet, 83(4), 417-425.

Srivastava, P., & Durgaprasad, S. (2008). Burn wound healing property of Cocos nucifera: An appraisal. Indian journal of pharmacology, 40(4), 144.

Molan, P. C. (2001). Potential of honey in the treatment of wounds and burns. American Journal of Clinical Dermatology, 2(1), 13-19.

Samuelsen, A. B. (2000). The traditional uses, chemical constituents and biological activities of Plantago major L. A review. Journal of ethnopharmacology, 71(1), 1-21.

Vakilian, K., Atarha, M., Bekhradi, R., & Chaman, R. (2011). Healing advantages of lavender essential oil during episiotomy recovery: a clinical trial. Complementary therapies in clinical practice, 17(1), 50-53.

Marshmallow. (n.d.). Retrieved July 23, 2016, from http://umm.edu/health/medical/altmed/herb/marshmallow

Koh, K. J., Pearce, A. L., Marshman, G., Finlay-Jones, J. J., & Hart, P. H. (2002). Tea tree oil reduces histamine-induced skin inflammation. British Journal of Dermatology, 147(6), 1212-1217.

Al-Howiriny, T. A., Al-Sohaibani, M. O., El-Tahir, K. H., & Rafatullah, S. (2003). Preliminary evaluation of the anti-inflammatory and anti-hepatotoxic activities of'parsley'petroselinum crispum in rats.

Ali, H. F., El-Beltagi, H. S., & Nasr, N. F. (2008). Assessment of volatile components, free radical-scavenging capacity and anti-microbial activity of Lemon verbena leaves. Research Journal of phytochemistry, 2(2), 84-92.

Aydin, A. A., Zerbes, V., Parlar, H., & Letzel, T. (2013, March 5). The medical plant butterbur (Petasites): Analytical and physiological (re)view. Journal of Pharmaceutical Biomedical Analysis, 75, 220-229. Retrieved fromhttp://www.ncbi.nlm.nih.gov/pubmed/23277154

Butterbur. (2016, January 5). Retrieved from https://nccih.nih.gov/health/butterburGuo, R., Pittler, M. H., & Ernst, E. (2007, December). Herbal medicines for the treatment of allergic rhinitis: a systematic review. Annal of Allergy, Asthma & Immunology, 99(6), 483-495. Retrieved fromhttp://www.ncbi.nlm.nih.gov/pubmed/18219828!

Aggarwal, Bharat B. "Potential Therapeutic Effects of Curcumin, the Anti-inflammatory Agent, Against Neurodegenerative, Cardiovascular, Pulmonary, Metabolic, Autoimmune and Neoplastic Diseases." Int J Biochem Cell Biol. 41. 1. (2009): 40-59. Web. June 4, 2016. http://www.ncbi.nlm.nih.gov/pmc/articles/PMC2637808/

Shin, H. S., See, H. J., Jung, S. Y., Choi, D. W., Kwon, D. A., Bae, M. J., ... & Shon, D. H. (2015). Turmeric (Curcuma longa) attenuates food allergy symptoms by regulating type 1/type 2 helper T cells (Th1/Th2) balance in a mouse model of food allergy. Journal of ethnopharmacology, 175, 21-29.

Babic, I., Nguyen-the, C., Amiot, M. J., & Aubert, S. (1994). Antimicrobial activity of shredded carrot extracts on food-borne bacteria and yeast. Journal of applied bacteriology, 76(2), 135-141.

Erickson, L. (2003). Rooibos tea: Research into antioxidant and antimutagenic properties. HerbalGram, 59, 34-45.

Srivastava, J. K., Shankar, E., & Gupta, S. (2010). Chamomile: A herbal medicine of the past with bright future. Molecular medicine reports, 3(6), 895.

Simon, A., Traynor, K., Santos, K., Blaser, G., Bode, U., & Molan, P. (2009). Medical honey for wound care—still the 'latest resort'?. Evidence-based complementary and alternative medicine, 6(2), 165-173.

Ernst, E., & Pittler, M. H. (2000). Efficacy of ginger for nausea and vomiting: a systematic review of randomized clinical trials. British journal of anaesthesia, 84(3), 367-371.

Korukluoglu, M., Sahan, Y., & Yigit, A. (2008). Antifungal properties of olive leaf extracts and their phenolic compounds. Journal of Food safety, 28(1), 76-87.